Endoscopic Mucosal Resection

Endoscopic Mucosal Resection

Edited by:

Massimo Conio, MD
Director, Department of Gastroenterology
   and Digestive Endoscopy
General Hospital
Sanremo (IM), Italy

Peter D. Siersema, MD, PhD
Professor of Gastroenterology
Director, Department of Gastroenterology
   and Hepatology, University Medical Center
Utrecht, The Netherlands

Alessandro Repici, MD
Director, Unit of Digestive Endoscopy Unit
Istituto Clinico Humanitas
Rozzano (MI), Italy

Thierry Ponchon, MD
Director, Department of Gastroenterology
Hôpital E. Herriot
Lyon, France

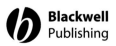
Blackwell
Publishing

Blackwell Publishing, Inc., 350 Main Street, Malden, Massachusetts 02148-5020, USA
Blackwell Publishing Ltd, 9600 Garsington Road, Oxford OX4 2DQ, UK
Blackwell Publishing Asia Pty Ltd, 550 Swanston Street, Carlton, Victoria 3053, Australia

First published 2008

1 2008

Library of Congress Cataloging-in-Publication Data
Endoscopic mucosal resection / edited by Massimo Conio ... [et al.].
    p. ; cm.
  Includes bibliographical references and index.
  ISBN 978-1-4051-5885-5 (alk. paper)
  1. Gastrointestinal system–Cancer–Endoscopic surgery. 2. Gastrointestinal mucosa–Endoscopic
surgery. I. Conio, Massimo.
  [DNLM: 1. Endoscopy, Digestive System–methods. 2. Gastric Mucosa–surgery. 3. Gastrointestinal
Neoplasms–surgery. 4. Intestinal Mucosa–surgery. WI 141 E543 2007]
  RD668.E53 2007
  616.99′433059--dc22
                                                          2007021141
  ISBN: 978-1-4051-5885-5

A catalogue record for this title is available from the British Library

Set in 10/13.5 Sabon by Newgen Imaging Systems (P) Ltd, Chennai, India
Printed and bound at GraphyCems, Navarra, Spain

Commissioning Editor: Alison Brown
Editorial Assistant: Jennifer Seward
Development Editors: Adam Gilbert and Victoria Pittman
Production Controller: Debbie Wyer

For further information on Blackwell Publishing, visit our website:
http://www.blackwellpublishing.com

The publisher's policy is to use permanent paper from mills that operate a sustainable forestry policy, and
which has been manufactured from pulp processed using acid-free and elementary chlorine-free practices.
Furthermore, the publisher ensures that the text paper and cover board used have met acceptable environmental accreditation standards.

Contents

List of Contributors

Pradeep Bhandari Solent Centre for Digestive Diseases, Portsmouth Hospital NHS Trust, Portsmouth, UK

Amitabh Chak, MD Professor of Medicine and Oncology, UH Case Medical Center, Case Western Reserve School of Medicine, Cleveland, OH, USA

Mihai Ciocirlan Department of Gastroenterology, Hôpital Edouard Herriot, Lyon, Frame

Jan-Willem W. Coebergh Comprehensive Cancer Centre South, Eindhoven Cancer Registry, Eindhoven, the Netherlands; Department of Public Health, Erasmus University Medical Center, Rotterdam, the Netherlands

Sergio Coda Operative Unit of Diagnostic and Therapeutic Endoscopy, Department of General and Specialized Surgery and Organ Transplantation "Paride Stefanini", University of Rome "La Sapienza", Rome, Italy

Salvatore Comunale Digestive Endoscopy Unit, IRCCS Istituto Clinico Humanitas, Milano, Italy

Massimo Conio Department of Gastroenterology and Digestive Endoscopy, General Hospital, Sanremo, Italy

Guido Costamagna Unità Operativa di Endoscopia Digestiva Chirurgica, Policlinico Universitario 'A.Gemelli', Università Cattolica del Sacro Cuore, Roma, Italy

Giuseppe De Caro Digestive Endoscopy Unit, IRCCS Istituto Clinico Humanitas, Milano, Italy

Christian Ell Department of Medicine II, HSK Wiesbaden, Teaching Hospital of the University of Mainz, Germany

Farees T. Farooq, MD, Fellow, Division of Gastroenterology, UH Case Medical Center, Case Western Reserve School of Medicine, Cleveland, OH, USA

Rosangela Filiberti Epidemiology and Biostatistics, National Cancer Research Institute, Genoa, Italy

Paul Fockens Department of Gastroenterology and Hepatology, Academic Medical Center, University of Amsterdam, Amsterdam, the Netherlands

Mitsuhiro Fujishiro The University of Tokyo Graduate School of Medicine, Tokyo, Japan

Liebwin Gossner Department of Internal Medicine I, Karlsruhe, Teaching Hospital of the University of Freiburg, Germany

Christopher Gostout Mayo Clinic Division of Gastroenterology and Hepatology, Rochester, MN, USA

Takuji Gotoda Head of Endoscopy Division, National Cancer Center Hospital, Tokyo, Japan

Keiichi Ikeda Department of Endoscopy, Jikei University School of Medicine, Tokyo, Japan

Hisatomo Ikehara Endoscopy Division, Shizuoka Cancer Center, Shizuoka, Japan

Naomi Kakushima Department of Gastroenterology, The University of Tokyo Graduate School of Medicine, Tokyo, Japan

Ralf Kiesslich Department of Internal Medicine, University of Mainz, Germany

Valery E.P.P. Lemmens Comprehensive Cancer Centre South, Eindhoven Cancer Registry, Eindhoven, the Netherlands; Department of Public Health, Erasmus University Medical Center, Rotterdam, the Netherlands

Carmelo Luigiano Digestive Endoscopy Unit, IRCCS Istituto Clinico Humanitas, Milano, Italy

Takahisa Matsuda Endoscopy Division, National Cancer Center Hospital, Tokyo, Japan

Helmut Messmann III Medical Department, Clinic of Augsburg, Augsburg, Germany

Ichiro Oda Endoscopy Division, National Cancer Center Hospital, Tokyo, Japan

Maria Antonietta Orengo Liguria Cancer Registry–Descriptive Epidemiology, National Cancer Research Institute, Genoa, Italy

Thierry Ponchon Department of Gastroenterology, Hôpital Edouard Herriot, Lyon, France

Alessandro Repici Digestive Endoscopy Unit, IRCCS Istituto Clinico Humanitas, Milano, Italy

Riccardo Rosati Mininvasive Surgical Unit, IRCCS Istituto Clinico Humanitas, Milano, Italy

Yutaka Saito Head of Endoscopy Divison, National Cancer Center Hospital, Tokyo, Japan

Peter D. Siersema Department of Gastroenterology and Hepatology, University Medical Center Utrecht, the Netherlands

Paul Swain Department of Surgical Oncology and Technology, Imperial College, St Mary's Hospital, London, UK

Kaiyo Takubo Department of Pathology, Tokyo Metropolitan Hospital, Tokyo, Japan

Michael Vieth Institute of Pathology, Klinikum Bayreuth, PreuschwitzerStr. 101, Bayreuth, Germany

Chizu Yokoi Endoscopy Division, National Cancer Center Hospital, Tokyo, Japan

Preface

Writing a book on any endotherapy subject also means accepting the fact that the concepts expressed have a high risk of aging rapidly. This risk is even higher when dealing with a technique which is still in evolution such as EMR. However, there is now a body of consolidated knowledge that can be used to promote a better endoscopy technique for EMR, even for endoscopists who are not familiar with this particular method.

This book is entirely dedicated to EMR, with the special purpose of discussing in detail the practical aspects of this new endotherapy technique. The EMR technique was introduced by Japanese endoscopists, and is now becoming increasingly popular in the West where the majority of endoscopists have no experience with this method. The impact of EMR in the clinical field has been tremendous, and now for a group of patients, when the removal of superficial cancers in the esophagus, stomach, duodenum and colorectum is indicated, open surgery can be avoided.

Up to now, EMR has been reported in journals devoted to endoscopy, such as *Gastrointestinal Endoscopy* or *Endoscopy*. A considerable number of articles have been published in these journals in the last two years on this procedure. Essential information about results and indications or when to apply this technique has been presented. However these articles do not consider the different scenarios in which the technique can be performed. Our book, which analyzes in depth the details of this technique, will likely fill this gap.

The purpose of the current book is to provide a careful step-by-step guide to aid the endoscopist in his daily clinical practice. Methods, details and particularities that are not usually reported in scientific articles have been described. A comprehensive and essential analysis of the literature has been included in each chapter, along with tables, diagrams and photographs to help the reader. All the technical aspects have been explained and clarified with high quality illustrations. Photographs of the available endoscopic devices have also been provided.

We wish to thank all the authors for their contribution to this book. They are all highly experienced endoscopists and well known at the international level. They have been able to condense their knowledge for these pages. A special thank you should also go to Blackwell Publishing for their excellent support.

We wish this book to be thought-provoking and hope that it stimulates new ideas and projects in the arena of therapeutic endoscopy, which has developed significantly over the last 10 years. New materials and accessories have aided the progressive diffusion of EMR and of endoscopic submuscosal dissection (ESD), even outside referral centres. We are certain that with the simplification of these methods, EMR and ESD will in the future be performed in most endoscopic departments worldwide.

We hope that this book can represent an important point of reference for those interested in this subject.

Massimo Conio, MD
Peter D. Siersema, MD
Alessandro Repici, MD
Thierry Ponchon, MD

Epidemiology of Gastrointestinal Cancer: (Trends in) Incidence and Mortality from Esophageal, Stomach, and Colorectal Cancer

VALERY E.P.P. LEMMENS AND JAN-WILLEM W. COEBERGH

Introduction

In the past decades, clinically and population-based studies in developed countries have reported increases in the incidence of adenocarcinoma of the esophagus, gastric cardia, and colorectum. This increase was not observed for squamous cell carcinoma of the esophagus and tumors of the non-gastric part of the stomach; the latter showed a clear decrease in incidence. A strong decrease in mortality from stomach cancer and a moderate decrease in mortality from colorectal cancer have been reported in several Western countries, while mortality rates increased for esophageal cancer. In developed countries, colorectal cancer has a higher incidence and mortality than esophageal and stomach cancer, while the opposite is true for less developed countries (Figs 1.1 and 1.2).

In this chapter, we will give an overview of the current incidence and mortality rates of esophageal, stomach, and colorectal cancer, including geographic variations and male–female differences. We will present the most important trends in time, with a more detailed view on trends in histology of esophageal and gastric cancer incidence and trends in subsite distribution of colorectal cancer incidence. We will discuss age-adjusted trends; it is important to bear in mind that even stable incidence rates can mean large increases in absolute numbers of newly diagnosed cancer patients in Western countries, due to the aging of the population.

Endoscopic Mucosal Resection. Edited by M. Conio, P. Siersema, A. Repici and T. Ponchon. © 2008 Blackwell Publishing. ISBN 978-1-4051-5885-5.

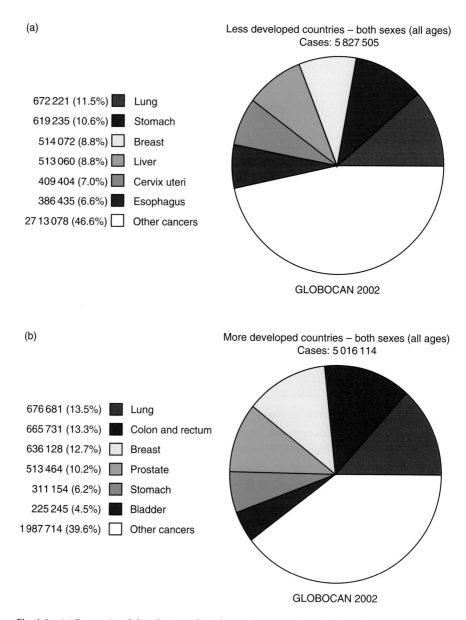

(a)

Less developed countries – both sexes (all ages)
Cases: 5 827 505

672 221 (11.5%) ■	Lung
619 235 (10.6%) ■	Stomach
514 072 (8.8%) □	Breast
513 060 (8.8%) ■	Liver
409 404 (7.0%) ■	Cervix uteri
386 435 (6.6%) ■	Esophagus
27 13 078 (46.6%) □	Other cancers

GLOBOCAN 2002

(b)

More developed countries – both sexes (all ages)
Cases: 5 016 114

676 681 (13.5%) ■	Lung
665 731 (13.3%) ■	Colon and rectum
636 128 (12.7%) □	Breast
513 464 (10.2%) ■	Prostate
311 154 (6.2%) ■	Stomach
225 245 (4.5%) ■	Bladder
1 987 714 (39.6%) □	Other cancers

GLOBOCAN 2002

Fig. 1.1   (a) Proportional distribution of incidence of cancer in less developed countries, in 2002.
(b) Proportional distribution of incidence of cancer in more developed countries, in 2002.

Methods

Esophageal, stomach, and colorectal cancer were classified according to the
International Classification of Disease (ICD, 10th revision): Esophagus (C15),
stomach (C16), and colon/rectum (C18–C21).

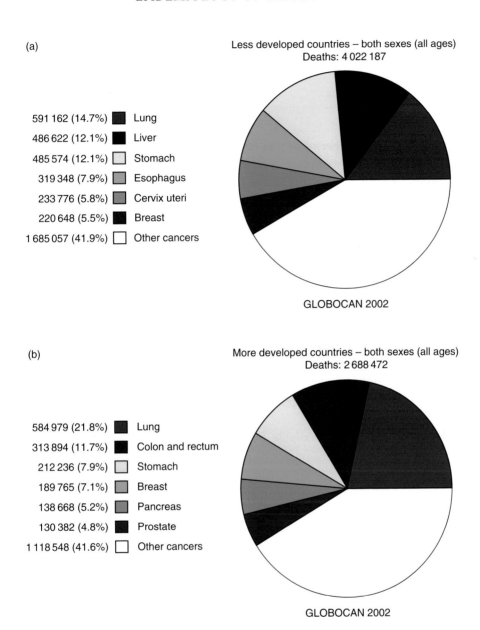

Fig. 1.2 (a) Proportional distribution of mortality from cancer in less developed countries, in 2002. (b) Proportional distribution of mortality from cancer in more developed countries, in 2002.

Incidence

Incidence is the number of new cases arising in a given period in a specified population. Cancer registries collect this information routinely. It can be expressed as an absolute number of cases per year or as a rate per 100 000 persons per year. The latter provides an approximation to the average risk of developing a cancer, which is particularly useful in making comparisons between populations.

Mortality

Mortality is the number of deaths occurring in a given period in a specified population. It can be expressed as an absolute number of deaths per year or as a rate per 100 000 persons per year.

Population

Estimates of the population of countries (by age and sex) for the year 2000 and 2005 were taken from the United Nations population projections (the 2002 revision). The population figures for the year 2002 were estimated by calculating the annual percentage change by sex and age between the year 2000 and 2005.

Analyses

All analyses were carried out using the GLOBOCAN software [1]. The GLOBOCAN 2002 database has been built up using the huge amount of data available in the Descriptive Epidemiology Group of the International Agency for Research on Cancer.

Incidence data were available from cancer registries. They cover entire national populations, or samples of such populations from selected regions. Cancer registries also provide statistics on cancer survival. With data on incidence, and on survival, we can estimate the prevalence of cancer (persons who are alive with cancer diagnosed within a given number of years of diagnosis). Mortality data by cause are available for many countries through the registration of vital events, although the degree of detail and quality of the data vary considerably. With such data, it is possible to prepare estimates of the numbers of new and prevalent cancer cases and deaths by site, sex, and age group. These are more or less accurate, for different countries, depending on the extent and accuracy of locally available data.

Age-standardized rate

All data are presented as standardized rates. An age-standardized rate (ASR) is a summary measure of a rate that a population would have if it had a standard age structure. The most frequently used standard population is the World standard population. The calculated incidence or mortality rate is then called the World age standardized incidence or mortality rate. It is expressed as a rate per 100 000.

Esophageal cancer

The incidence of esophageal cancer in 2002 was particularly high in Western Europe, south-central Asia, eastern Africa, and parts of South America (Figs 1.3 and 1.4). It was lowest in western Africa and in Indonesia. This pattern was equal for both males and females. In the developed countries, the incidence of esophageal cancer was the highest in the United Kingdom, France, Ireland, and Japan, and lowest in Norway, Finland, and Malta (Fig. 1.5). The incidence in males was much larger than in females, this difference was largest in France and Slovakia.

In countries with a high incidence of esophageal cancer, such as Japan and the United Kingdom, the incidence was especially high among elderly people (Fig. 1.6).

There has been a large increase of adenocarcinoma of the esophagus in many developed countries, compared with a decrease of squamous cell carcinoma. Rates of adenocarcinoma have been increasing in the USA, United Kingdom, Scandinavia, France, Switzerland, Denmark, Italy, Slovakia, the Netherlands (restricted to males), Australia, and New Zealand [2–4]. This might be partly due to a diagnostic shift; tumors arising in the cardio-esophageal junction are classified with gastric cardia tumors; an increase in esophageal adenocarcinoma

Incidence of esophageal cancer: ASR (World) – Male (all ages)

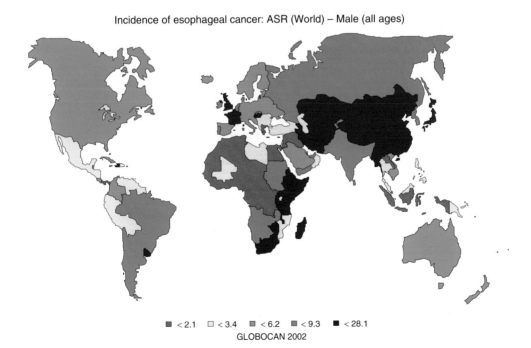

■ < 2.1   □ < 3.4   ■ < 6.2   ■ < 9.3   ■ < 28.1
GLOBOCAN 2002

Fig. 1.3 Incidence of esophageal cancer in males, 2002, worldwide.

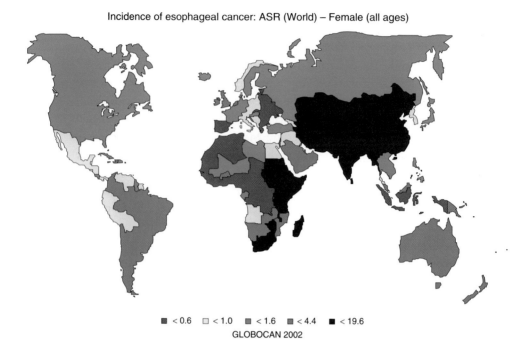

Fig. 1.4   Incidence of esophageal cancer in females, 2002, worldwide.

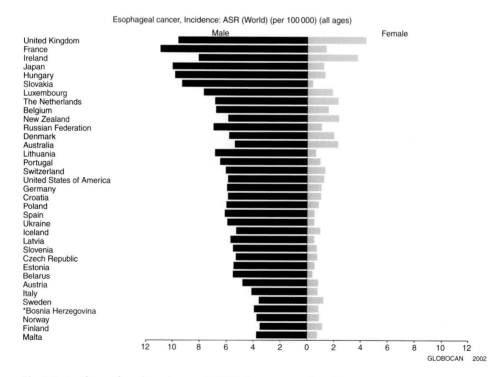

Fig. 1.5   Incidence of esophageal cancer in 2002, by country and gender.

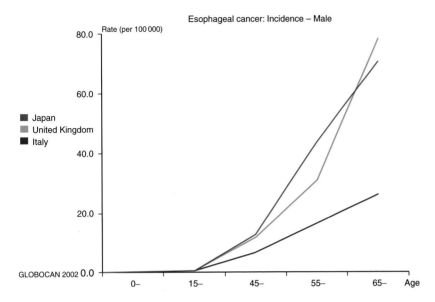

Fig. 1.6 Incidence of esophageal cancer in 2002, by age, among males in three selected countries.

could appear if tumors at or near the junction were identified increasingly as being esophageal in origin. However, gastric cardia rates would then diminish to a similar extent, which has not occurred. Rates may increase with earlier endoscopy-based diagnosis, but the stage distribution has not changed over time, and survival consistently has been poor, even for patients diagnosed with localized disease. These observations suggest that the increase of adenocarcinoma of the esophagus is real and reflects changes in the prevalence of risk factors [2].

Mortality from esophageal cancer showed the same patterns as the incidence (Figs 1.7, 1.8, and 1.9). Due to the increased incidence and the very limited improvements in survival of people with esophageal cancer, mortality rates have been increasing in most countries.

Stomach cancer

The incidence of stomach cancer in 2002 was highest in northern Asia, including China and Japan, eastern Europe, southern Europe, and eastern South America. Lowest rates were found in Africa and Indonesia (Figs 1.10 and 1.11). Among developed countries, rates were by far the highest in Japan, and lowest in the USA (Fig. 1.12). Stomach cancer was more common among males than among females. Already by middle age, in Japan the incidence of stomach cancer is much higher compared to, for example, the USA or Italy (Fig. 1.13).

While there has been a marked decline in distal, intestinal-type gastric cancers (especially among females), the incidence of proximal, diffuse-type

Mortality from esophageal cancer: ASR (World) – Male (all ages)

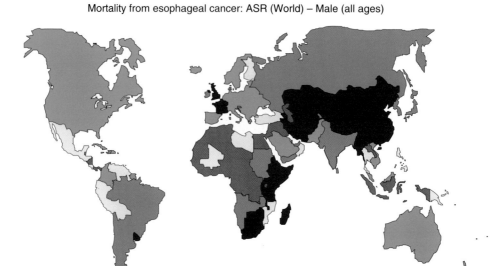

■ < 1.9   □ < 3.0   ■ < 5.7   ■ < 8.6   ■ < 27.4
GLOBOCAN 2002

Fig. 1.7   Mortality from esophageal cancer in males, 2002, worldwide.

Incidence of esophageal cancer: ASR (World) – Female (all ages)

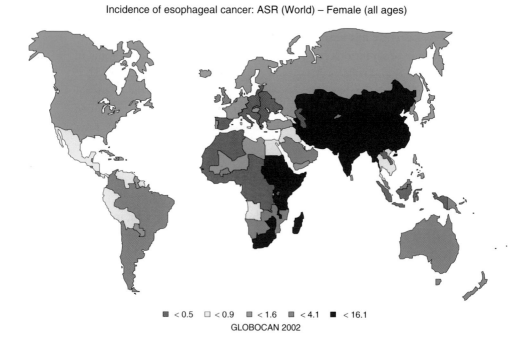

■ < 0.5   □ < 0.9   ■ < 1.6   ■ < 4.1   ■ < 16.1
GLOBOCAN 2002

Fig. 1.8   Mortality from esophageal cancer in females, 2002, worldwide.

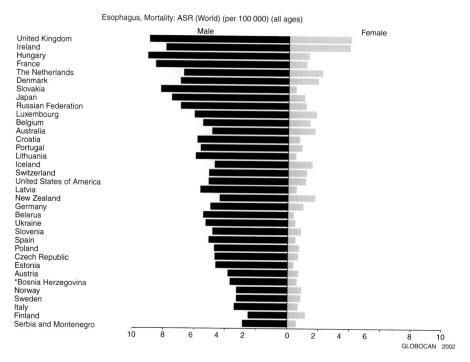

Fig. 1.9 Mortality from esophageal cancer, 2002, by country and gender.

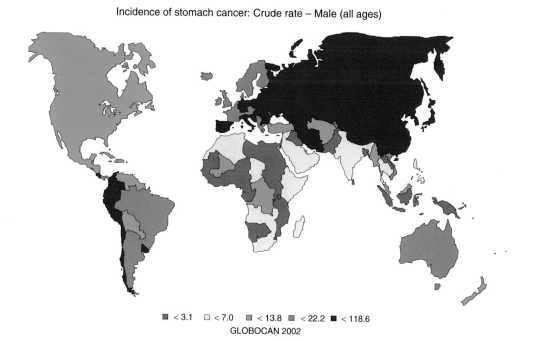

Fig. 1.10 Incidence of stomach cancer in males, 2002, worldwide.

Incidence of stomach cancer: Crude rate – Female (all ages)

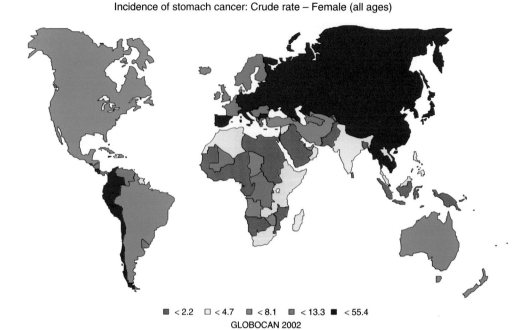

■ < 2.2   □ < 4.7   ▨ < 8.1   ▦ < 13.3   ■ < 55.4

GLOBOCAN 2002

Fig. 1.11   Incidence of stomach cancer in females, 2002, worldwide.

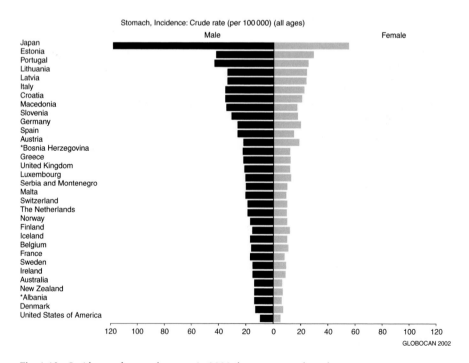

Fig. 1.12   Incidence of stomach cancer in 2002, by country and gender.

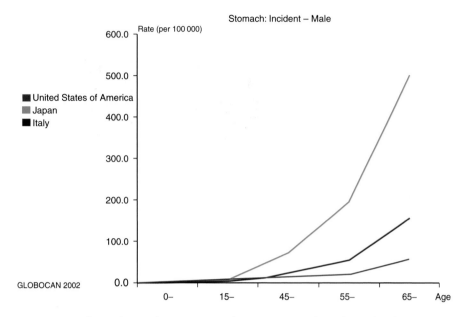

Fig. 1.13 Incidence of stomach cancer in 2002, by age, among males in three selected countries.

adenocarcinomas of the gastric cardia has been increasing, particularly in Western countries. Incidence by tumor subsite also varies widely based on geographic location, race, and socio-economic status. Distal gastric cancer predominates in developing countries, among black people, and in lower socio-economic groups, whereas proximal tumors are more common in developed countries, among white people, and in higher socio-economic classes. Diverging trends in the incidence of gastric cancer by tumor location suggest that they may represent two diseases with different etiologies [5].

Over the past few years, gastric cancer mortality has decreased markedly in most areas of the world. However, gastric cancer remains a disease of high mortality, second only to lung cancer as the leading cause of cancer-related death worldwide (Figs 1.14 and 1.15).

Availability of screening for early detection in high-risk areas has led to a decrease in mortality. In Japan, mortality rates for gastric cancer in men have halved since the introduction of screening in the 1970s [5]. Mortality rates in 2002 were lower in Japan than in some eastern European countries (Fig. 1.16).

Colorectal cancer

The incidence of colorectal cancer showed a different picture than the incidence of esophageal or stomach cancer. Colorectal cancer is predominantly a cancer

Mortality from stomach cancer: ASR (World) – Male (all ages)

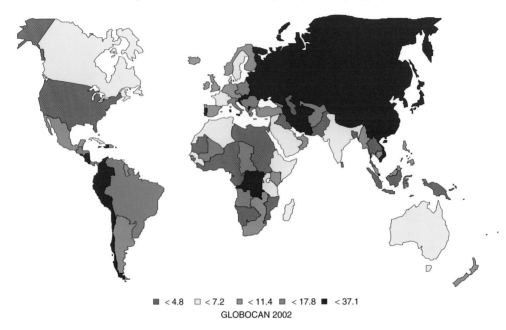

■ < 4.8   □ < 7.2   ■ < 11.4   ■ < 17.8   ■ < 37.1
GLOBOCAN 2002

Fig. 1.14   Mortality from stomach cancer in males, 2002, worldwide.

Mortality from stomach cancer: ASR (World – Female (all ages)

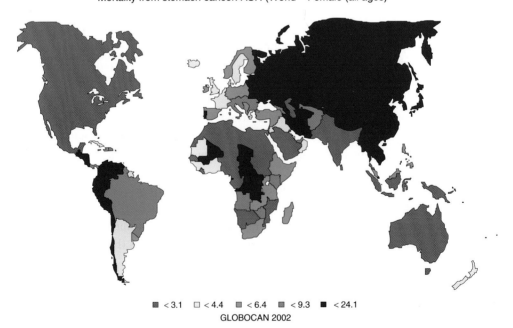

■ < 3.1   □ < 4.4   ■ < 6.4   ■ < 9.3   ■ < 24.1
GLOBOCAN 2002

Fig. 1.15   Mortality from stomach cancer in females, 2002, worldwide.

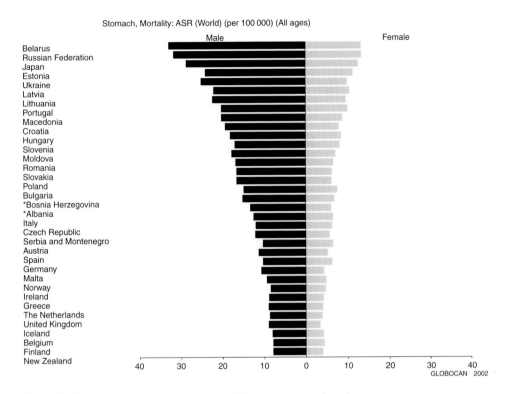

Fig. 1.16 Mortality from stomach cancer in 2002, by country and gender.

of the developed world. It was most common in 2002 in Europe, the USA, and Australia, for both males and females (Figs 1.17 and 1.18). It was somewhat more frequent among males than among females. The highest incidence was found in Germany, Hungary, Japan (especially males), the Czech Republic, and Norway (especially females), while the lowest rates in the Western world were found in the Ukraine and in Greece (Fig. 1.19).

Colorectal cancer in all countries is predominantly a disease of elderly people.

While the incidence rates in the USA and Canada have been stable for two decades, incidence is still increasing in many European countries, especially among men. In many countries, a shift toward more proximal tumors has been noted [6–10]. Exposure to changing risk factors is probably the cause of this shift. Also the male-to-female rate ratio progressively increased from the proximal colon to the distal colorectum, and the ratio of proximal-to-distal colorectal cancer gradually increased with advancing age [11].

Colorectal cancer mortality showed the same patterns as colorectal incidence (Figs 1.20 and 1.21). Mortality was highest in Hungary, the Czech Republic, and Slovakia (Fig. 1.22). A favorable pattern in colorectal cancer mortality for both genders was observed in most European countries from the 1990s onward.

Incidence of colon and rectum cancer: Crude rate – Male (all ages)

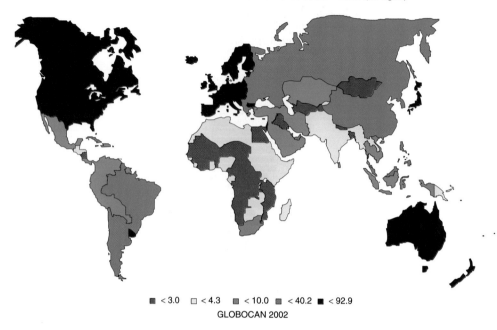

■ < 3.0   □ < 4.3   ■ < 10.0   ■ < 40.2   ■ < 92.9
GLOBOCAN 2002

Fig. 1.17   Incidence of colorectal cancer in males, 2002, worldwide.

Incidence of colon and rectum cancer: Crude rate – Female (all ages)

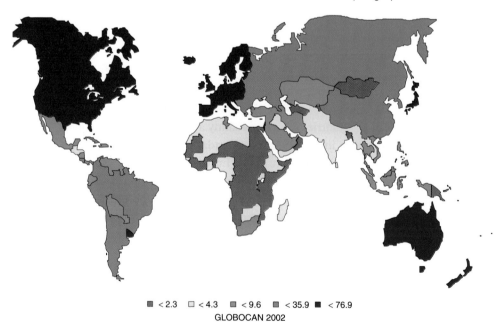

■ < 2.3   □ < 4.3   ■ < 9.6   ■ < 35.9   ■ < 76.9
GLOBOCAN 2002

Fig. 1.18   Incidence of colorectal cancer in females, 2002, worldwide.

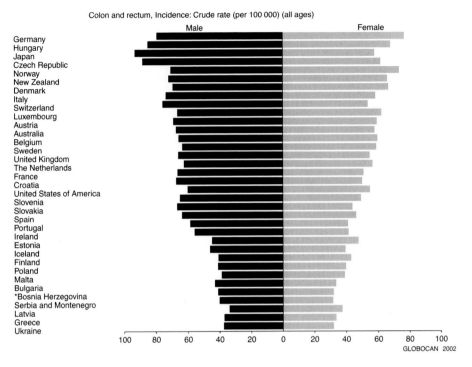

Fig. 1.19   Incidence of colorectal cancer in 2002, by country and gender.

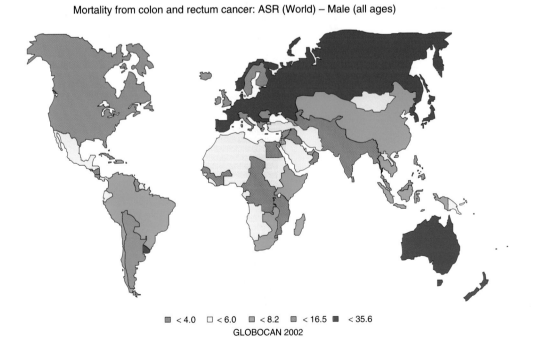

Fig. 1.20   Mortality from colorectal cancer in males, 2002, worldwide.

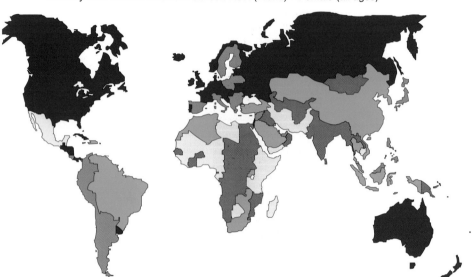

Mortality from colon and rectum cancer: ASR (World) – Female (all ages)

■ < 3.0   □ < 4.4   ■ < 7.2   ■ < 11.5   ■ < 21.2

GLOBOCAN 2002

Fig. 1.21 Mortality from colorectal cancer in females, 2002, worldwide.

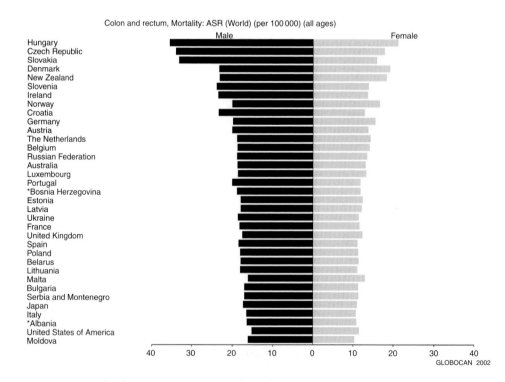

Fig. 1.22 Mortality from colorectal cancer in 2002, by country and gender.

Lower incidence rates, earlier detection, and improvements in treatment were responsible for this. Colorectal cancer mortality rates were still in the upward direction in some eastern European countries, as well as in some Mediterranean countries. Mortality rates tended to converge, a pattern even clearer when colorectal mortality rates were examined in three broad European regions. Similar mortality rates over recent calendar years have been reached by countries where mortality has been decreasing in recent decades, and in those countries (mainly eastern European and Mediterranean countries) which have experienced a recent leveling-off and decrease [12].

References

1 Ferlay J, Bray F, Pisani P, Parkin M. GLOBOCAN 2002 Cancer Incidence, Mortality and Prevalence Worldwide. IARC Press, Lyon, 2004.
2 Devesa SS, Blot WJ, Fraumeni JF, Jr. Changing patterns in the incidence of esophageal and gastric carcinoma in the United States. Cancer 1998; 83(10): 2049–53.
3 Botterweck AA, Schouten LJ, Volovics A, Dorant E, van Den Brandt PA. Trends in incidence of adenocarcinoma of the oesophagus and gastric cardia in ten European countries. Int J Epidemiol 2000; 29(4): 645–54.
4 Wijnhoven BP, Louwman MW, Tilanus HW, Coebergh JW. Increased incidence of adenocarcinomas at the gastro-oesophageal junction in Dutch males since the 1990s. Eur J Gastroenterol Hepatol 2002; 14(2): 115–22.
5 Crew KD, Neugut AI. Epidemiology of gastric cancer. World J Gastroenterol 2006; 12(3): 354–62.
6 Svensson E, Grotmol T, Hoff G, Langmark F, Norstein J, Tretli S. Trends in colorectal cancer incidence in Norway by gender and anatomic site: an age-period-cohort analysis. Eur J Cancer Prev 2002; 11(5): 489–95.
7 Nelson RL, Persky V, Turyk M. Carcinoma in situ of the colorectum: SEER trends by race, gender, and total colorectal cancer. J Surg Oncol 1999; 71(2): 123–9.
8 Miller A, Gorska M, Bassett M. Proximal shift of colorectal cancer in the Australian Capital Territory over 20 years. Aust N Z J Med 2000; 30(2): 221–5.
9 Gibbons L, Waters C, Mao Y, Ellison L. Trends in colorectal cancer incidence and mortality. Health Rep 2001; 12(2): 41–55.
10 Cucino C, Buchner AM, Sonnenberg A. Continued rightward shift of colorectal cancer. Dis Colon Rectum 2002; 45(8): 1035–40.
11 Cheng X, Chen VW, Steele B et al. Subsite-specific incidence rate and stage of disease in colorectal cancer by race, gender, and age group in the United States, 1992–1997. Cancer 2001; 92(10): 2547–54.
12 Fernandez E, La Vecchia C, Gonzalez JR, Lucchini F, Negri E, Levi F. Converging patterns of colorectal cancer mortality in Europe. Eur J Cancer 2005; 41(3): 430–7.

CHAPTER 2

Etiological Factors in Gastrointestinal Tumors

ROSANGELA FILIBERTI AND MARIA ANTONIETTA ORENGO

Introduction

The etiology of gastrointestinal cancers is multifactorial, and differences in the exposure to a range of environmental factors account for much of the variation seen in the incidence of these tumors over time and among populations. However, so far it has not been clear to what extent the risk is due to the environment or to genetic factors, and studies are now focusing on the interaction between exogenous factors and individual susceptibility.

This chapter will focus on esophageal, gastric, and colorectal cancers and will give an overall outlook on epidemiologic findings about these pathologies. In Tables 2.1–2.5 a selection of studies on some factors involved in the etiology of these diseases is reported.

Esophageal cancers

The increasing incidence trends observed for adenocarcinomas of the esophagus (EA) in Western countries, associated with stable or declining incidence trends for esophageal squamous cell carcinoma (ESCC), suggest that different risk factors may be associated with these tumors. The improvement of different diagnostic and/or classification criteria, as well as the changes in time of the histological confirmation, can only partially explain the observed trends.

Esophageal squamous cell carcinoma

ESCC often arises from preceding dysplastic lesions in the esophageal epithelium and DNA methylation appears to contribute to the progression of dysplasia–carcinoma sequence [1].

Endoscopic Mucosal Resection. Edited by M. Conio, P. Siersema, A. Repici and T. Ponchon. © 2008 Blackwell Publishing. ISBN 978-1-4051-5885-5.

Table 2.1   Smoking and gastrointestinal tumors.

Cancer	Author	RR and their 95% confidence intervals
Esophageal AC	Gammon et al., 1997 [23] (C–C) (293 cancers – 695 controls)	2.2 (1.4–3.3)
	Wu et al., 2001 [20] (C–C) (222 cancers –1356 controls)	2.8 (1.8–4.3)
Esophageal squamous cell carcinoma	Gallus et al., 2003 [84] (C–C) (395 cancers – 1006 controls) Zambon et al., 2000 [2] (C–C) (275 cancers – 593 controls)	<20 mg tar: 4.8 (3.1–7.6) ≥20 mg tar: 5.4 (3.2–9.3) ≥25 cigarettes/day: 7.0 (3.2–15.1) Smoking for ≥35 years: 6.4 (3.5–12.0)
Cardia AC	Wu et al., 2001 [20] (C–C) (277 cancers – 1356 controls)	2.12 (1.5–3.1)
Distal gastric AC	Wu et al., 2001 [20] (C–C) (443 cancers – 1356 controls)	1.5 (1.1–2.1)
Gastric AC	Sasazuki et al., 2002 [85] (Cohort, 293 cancers)	2.1 (1.2–3.6)
	Fujino et al., 2005 [86] (Cohort, 757 cancers)	1.36 (1.07–1.73)
Colorectal AC	Verla-Tebit et al., 2006 [62] (C–C) (540 cancers – 614 controls)	Smoking ≥30 years: 1.25 (0.90–1.75) Smoking ≥40 pack-years: 1.92 (1.13–3.28) Quitting smoking ≥40 years vs. current smokers: 0 .46 (0.21–0.98)
	Limburg et al., 2003 [87] (Cohort, 41 836 women – 1118 cancers)	1.17 (1.00–1.36)

AC: adenocarcinoma; C–C: case–control study; RR: relative risk point estimates for smokers vs. non-smokers.

Table 2.2   Obesity, glycemic profile, physical activity, and gastrointestinal tumors.

Cancer	Author	RR and their 95% confidence intervals
Esophageal AC	Lindblad et al., 2005 [19] (C–C nested) (287 cancers – 10 000 controls)	BMI >25 kg/m^2: 1.67 (1.22–2.30)
	Engeland et al., 2004 [88] (Cohort, 2245 cancers)	BMI ≥30 kg/m^2: 2.58 (1.81–3.68) men 2.06 (1.25–3.39) women
	Vigen et al., 2006 [89] (C–C) (212 cancers – 1330 controls)	Mean annual activity index: highest vs. lowest quartile: 0.61 (0.38–0.99)

Continued

Table 2.2 (*Continued*)

Cancer	Author	RR and their 95% confidence intervals
Esophageal AC	Kubo *et al.*, 2006 [90] Meta-analysis: 2488 cancers	BMI >25 kg/m²: 2.2 (1.7–2.7) men BMI >25 kg/m²: 2.0 (1.4–2.9) women
Esophageal squamous cells carcinoma	Engeland *et al.*, 2004 [88] (Cohort, 2245 cancers)	BMI ≥30 kg/m²: 0.68 (0.5–0.93) men 0.43 (0.32–0.59) women
Cardia AC	Lindblad *et al.*, 2005 [19] (C–C nested) (195 cancers – 10 000 controls) Vigen *et al.*, 2006 [89] (C–C) (264 cancers – 1330 controls)	BMI >25 kg/m²: 1.46 (0.98–2.18) Mean annual activity index: highest vs. lowest quartile: 0.76 (0.49–1.18)
Distal gastric AC	Lindblad *et al.*, 2005 [19] (C–C nested) (327 cancers – 10 000 controls) Vigen *et al.*, 2006 [89] (C–C) (389 cancers – 1330 controls)	BMI >25 kg/m²: no association Mean annual activity index: highest vs. lowest quartile: 0.77 (0.52–1.14)
Colorectal AC	Engeland *et al.*, 2005 [63] (Cohort, 47 117 cancers) Lin *et al.*, 2004 [91] (Cohort, 202 cancers in women) Franceschi *et al.*, 2001 [92] (C–C) (2953 cancers – 4154 controls) McCarl *et al.*, 2006 [69] (Cohort, 954 cancers)	Height 10 cm increase: 1.14 (1.11–1.16) men; 1.17(1.14–1.20) women BMI = 27–29.9 kg/m²: 1.72 (1.12–2.66) BMI ≥30 kg/m² vs. BMI <23 kg/m²: 1.67 (1.08–2.59) GI highest vs. lowest quintile: 1.7(1.4–2.0) In obese women: GI highest vs. lowest quintile: 1.66 (1.13–2.43) GL highest vs. lowest quintile: 1.79 (1.19–2.70)
Rectal AC	Mao *et al.*, 2003 [93] (C–C) (1447 cancers – 3106 controls)	Caloric intake: highest vs. lowest quartile: 1.61 (1.12–2.28) men BMI ≥30 kg/m²: 1.78 (1.36–2.34) men Caloric intake: highest vs. lowest quartile: 1.50 (1.00–2.28) women BMI ≥30 kg/m²: 1.44 (1.06–1.95) women

AC: adenocarcinoma; BMI: body mass index; C–C: case–control study; GI: glycemic index, GL: glycemic load; RR: relative risk point estimates.

Table 2.3   Pathological conditions related to esophageal and gastric tumors.

Cancer	Author	RR and their 95% confidence intervals
Esophageal AC	Wu *et al.*, 2003 [10] (C–C) (222 cancers – 1356 controls)	GERD: 3.61 (2.49–5.25) Hiatal hernia: 5.85 (3.18–10.75) GERD + Hiatal hernia: 8.11 (4.75–3.87)
	Farrow *et al.*, 2006 [9] (C–C) (293 cancers – 695 controls)	GERD daily symptoms: 5.5 (3.2–9.3)
	Ye *et al.*, 2004 [16] (C–C) (97 cancers – 499 controls)	*Hp* CagA+: 0.5 (0.3–0.8) Gastric atrophy: 1.1 (0.5–2.5)
Esophageal squamous cell carcinoma	Farrow *et al.*, 2006 [9] (C–C) (221 cancers – 695 controls)	GERD: no association
	Ye *et al.*, 2004 [16] (C–C) (85 cancers – 499 controls)	*Hp* CagA+: 2.1 (1.1–4.0) Gastric atrophy: 4.3 (1.9–9.6)
Cardia AC	Wu *et al.*, 2003 [17] (C–C) (87 cancers – 356 controls)	Seropositivity for *Hp*: 1.26 (0.82–1.94)
	Farrow *et al.*, 2006 [9] (C–C) (261 cancers – 695 controls)	GERD: no association
	Ye *et al.*, 2004 [16] (C–C) (133 cancers – 499 controls)	*Hp* CagA+: no association Gastric atrophy: 4.5 (2.5–7.8)
	Kamangar *et al.*, 2006 [34] (C–C) (61 cancers – 234 controls)	*Hp* CagA+: 0.31 (0.11–0.89)
Distal gastric AC	Wu *et al.*, 2003 [10] (C–C) (127 cancers – 356 controls)	Seropositivity for *Hp*: 1.85 (1.03–3.32)
	Farrow *et al.*, 2006 [9] (C–C) (368 cancers – 695 controls)	GERD: no association
	Knekt *et al.*, 2006 [33] (C–C nested) (225 cancers – 435 controls) – *Hp* infected vs. no infected	High IgA: 3.12 (1.97–4.95) High IgG: 2.88 (1.63–5.07) High IgA and Ig G, low PGI: 10.9 (4.31–27.7) vs. negative antibody and normal PGI
	Kamangar *et al.*, 2006 [33] (C–C) (173 cancers – 234 controls)	*Hp* CagA+: 7.9 (3.0–20.9)

AC: adenocarcinoma; C–C: case–controls; GERD: gastroesophageal reflux disease; *Hp*: *helicobacter pylori* infection; PGI: serum pepsinogen I; RR: relative risk point estimates.

In Western areas tobacco and alcohol may be responsible for more than 80% of cases. Forty-five per cent of tumors may be due to elevated alcohol use [2,3]. A case-control performed in northern Italy, in an area where heavy alcohol consumption is common, showed that, when considering exposure intensity, the risk from alchool was higher than the one from smoking. In addition, the association between high levels of smoking and alcohol consumption increased the risk by 130 times [2].

Table 2.4 Risk or protective dietary factors and gastroesophageal tumors.

Cancer	Author	RR and their 95% confidence intervals
Esophageal AC	Bahmanyar, 2006 [3] (C–C) (185 cancers – 815 controls)	Western diet (high 3rd tertile vs. lowest 1st tertile): 1.6 (0.9–3.1)
Esophageal squamous cell carcinoma	Bollschweiler et al., 2002 [94] (C–C) (52 cancers – 50 controls)	Vit. E intake >13 mg/day: 0.13 (0.1–0.5) Vit. C intake >100 mg/day: 0.33 (0.11–0.92)
	De Stefani et al., 2003 [7] (C–C) (116 cancers – 664 controls)	Red meat: 2.4 (1.4–4.2) White meat: 0.5 (0.3–0.9) Fruit: 0.2 (0.1–0.4) Vegetables: 0.7 (0.4–1.2)
	De Stefani et al., 2005 [4] (C–C) (200 cancers – 400 controls)	Total fruit: 0.48 (0.35–0.66) Citrus fruit: 0.47 (0.34–0.67)
Cardia AC	Bahmanyar, 2006 [3] (C–C) (258 cancers – 815 controls)	Western diet (high 3rd tertile vs. lowest 1st quartile): 1.8 (1.1–2.9)
	Zambon et al., 2000 [2] (C–C) (275 cancers – 593 controls)	35–55 alcohol drinks per week vs. light drinkers: 6.2 (3.2–2.2) 84 or more alcohol drinks per week vs. light drinkers: 24.5 (11.7–51.0)
Distal gastric AC	Gonzalez et al., 2006 [31] (Cohort, 330 cancers)	Total meat 100 g/day increase: 3.52 (1.96–6.34) Red meat 50 g/day increase: 1.73 (1.03–2.88) Processed meat 50 g/day increase: 2.45 (1.43–4.21) Total meat + Hp:5.32 (2.10–13.4)
Gastric AC	Kobayashi et al., 2002 [95] (Cohort, 404 cancers)	Vegetables ≥1 day/week Yellow vegetables: 0.64 (0.45–0.92) White vegetables: 0.48 (0.25–0.89) Fruits ≥1 day/week: 0.70 (0.49–1.0)
	Larsson et al., 2006 [96] (Cohort, 156 cancers)	All processed meat: Highest vs. lowest intake: 1.66 (1.13–2.45) Bacon or side pork: 1.55 (1.00–2.41) N-nitrosodimethylamine high quintile vs. lowest: 1.96 (1.08–3.58)

AC: adenocarcinoma; C–C: case–control study; Hp: *helicobacter pylori* infection; RR: relative risk point estimates; Western diet: high in processed meat, red meat, sweets, high-fat dairy, high-fat gravy.

Table 2.5 Risk or protective factors and colorectal tumors.

Cancer	Author	RR and their 95% confidence intervals
Colorectal AC	Norat et al., 2005 [48] (Cohort, 1329 cancers)	Red and processed meat: >160 g/day vs. <20 g/day: 1.35 (0.96–1.88) Fish: >80 g/day vs. <10 g/day: 0.69 (0.54–0.88)
	Larsson et al., 2006 [55] (Cohort, 449 cancers in men)	Total calcium: highest quartile vs. lowest quartile: 0.68 (0.51–0.91) Dairy foods: ≥7servings/day vs. <2 servings/day: 0.46 (0.30–0.71)
	Lin et al., 2005 [97] (Cohort, women, 223 cancers)	Fruit: highest vs. lowest quintile: 0.79 (0.49–1.27) Vegetables: highest vs. lowest quintile: 0.88 (0.56–1.38) Total fiber: highest vs. lowest quintile: 0.75 (0.48–1.17) Legume fiber: highest vs. lowest quintile: 0.60 (0.40–0.91)
	Larsson et al., 2005 [98] (Cohort, 805 colorectal cancers)	Dietary Folate intake: highest vs. lowest quintile: 0.61 (0.41–0.91) for colon cancers Dietary Folate intake: highest vs. lowest quintile: 0.93 (0.55–1.56) for rectal cancers
	Nichols et al., 2005 [73] (C–C) (1122 colon and 326 rectal cancers; 4297 controls)	OC users vs. never users: 0.89 (0.75–1.06) Premenopausal women vs. postmenopausal women: 0.67 (0.47–0.97) Recent OC users vs. never users: 0.53 (0.28–1.00) Five or more births vs. nulliparous: 0.66 (0.43–1.02) Women with age at first birth older than the median vs. age at first birth below the median: 0.83 (0.70–0.98)
	Larsson and Wolk, 2006 [99] Meta-analysis: Studies on red meat: 7367 cancers Studies on processed meat: 7903 cancers	Highest vs. lowest intake red meat: 1.28 (1.15–1.42) Highest vs. lowest intake processed meat: 1.20 (1.11–1.31)

AC: adenocarcinoma; C–C: case–control study; OC: oral contraceptives; RR: relative risk point estimates.

Dietary factors are considered important in the prevention of ESCC. A protective effect is attributed to fruit and vegetables and a 40% lower risk is associated with an intake of about five servings/day [4,5]. Protection is conferred partly through an antioxidative mechanism. With regard to nutrients, an inverse association was found for fiber, β-carotene, folate, vitamin C, and vitamin B6 [6]. Foods ingested at high temperature, such as stewed meat, could be a risk factor for ESCC [7]. It could be said that elimination of smoking, reduction of alcohol consumption, and enrichment of the diet with fruit and vegetables would make esophageal cancer a rare disease in Western areas.

Esophageal adenocarcinoma

In an analysis of national population-based incidence data from Italy, we found a significant upward trend for EA in males over the age of 60 years. The adenocarcinomas of the junction, conventionally classified by cancer registries as cardia tumors, increased in older males and also in younger females. It is still controversial whether EA and cardia adenocarcinoma represent a unique entity [8].

The etiology of EA is dominated by non-genetic risk factors, but so far the epidemiology of this cancer has not yet been solved and it is still uncertain which factors cause the increasing incidence. Gastroesophageal reflux (GERD) is an established risk factor for EA. The more frequent, more severe, and longer lasting the symptoms of reflux, the greater the risk. The use of medications that relax the lower esophageal sphincter might contribute to increasing the risk facilitating the reflux [9,10].

In recent years, attention has been focused on Barrett's esophagus (BE) and on the BE-dysplasia-adenocarcinoma sequence. BE is an acquired condition secondary to longstanding GERD [9]. It is present in about 5–10% of patients having endoscopy for reflux symptoms and is more likely to be present in obese people [11]. BE is considered to be a precancerous lesion and a strong risk factor for EA and, to a lesser extent, for cardia adenocarcinoma. Recent studies estimated an incidence of one adenocarcinoma for every 200 to 220 patients with BE per year [12]. People with BE have an excess risk of developing adenocarcinoma 30- to 125-fold relative to the risk of the general population [13]. In the few reported long-term surveillance studies the incidence of EA in high-grade dysplasia patients was 16–26% [12]. Nevertheless, among patients presenting with EA in a previously undiagnosed BE, only about 60% had chronic reflux symptoms. In a study on a Swedish population undergoing endoscopy, BE was present in 2% of participants. Overall, 40% reported reflux symptoms and 15% showed esophagitis. The prevalence of BE was 2% and 1% in people with and without GERD, respectively [14].

Evidence of an inverse relation between *Helicobacter pylori* (*Hp*) infection and risk of EA is getting stronger, suggesting that *Hp* may decrease the risk of EA by 50–80% [15,16], but more studies are warranted to establish these findings [17].

There are few known dietary risk factors. The best established risk exposure is a low intake of fruit, vegetables and fibers and, in particular, of antioxidants [5,6,18]. Other potential dietary risk factors include high intake of dietary fat, dietary cholesterol, and animal protein [6].

There are strong indications that there is a dose dependent association between increasing BMI and risk of EA [19,20]. EA patients and refluxers had a significantly higher BMI than patients with ESCC. The contribution of obesity, as well as of reflux, in explaining the increasing incidence of EA is unclear, because the prevalence trends of these two factors do not match those of EA incidence [21].

Tobacco smoking is a controversial issue and any association with smoking seems to be of moderate importance [22]. In studies in which a significant increase of risk for smokers emerged, it was suggested that the shift in esophageal histology could be mostly due to changes in tobacco constituents [20,23]. Alcohol consumption is not a risk factor, independent of the type of alcoholic beverage consumed [20,24].

Several studies have indicated an anti-tumoral effect with the use of non-steroidal anti-inflammatory drugs (NSAIDs), especially by using selective cyclooxygenase-2 inhibitors [25].

Gastric adenocarcinoma

Data from medical literature show that the two major histopathological variants in gastric adenocarcinoma (GA) are associated with a different distribution and different etiologic factors. The diffuse type occurs more often in young patients [26], it is more likely to have a primary genetic etiology and is not associated with intestinal metaplasia [27].

The intestinal type cancers are more frequently sporadic and associated with environmental factors. They may arise from chronic atrophic gastritis, which has a prevalence in gastroscopies of 28% (severe 8%) [28,29]. Gastric carcinogenesis is a continuous process from non-atrophic gastritis to glandular atrophy, to metaplasia and dysplasia, and to adenocarcinoma. Foods rich in salt; smoked or poorly preserved foods; and processed meat can induce atrophic gastritis and generate carcinogenic N-nitroso compounds in the gastric environment [30]. The association with red meat intake seems to be present for non-cardia adenocarcinoma (NCA), especially in people who were *Hp* antibody-positive, but not for cardia adenocarcinoma (CA) [31].

The association between *Hp* infection and GA has been postulated by independent studies indicating that *Hp* plays a dual role in the etiology of different gastric subsites. A prolonged infection with *Hp* (more than 10 years) seems to double the risk of NCA, mainly of intestinal-type [32,33], but is inversely associated with the risk of CA [34]. An increased risk of NCA has also been associated with a history of gastric ulcer [9].

The role of environmental factors in the etiology of GA was suggested in the late 1960s by studies on migrants from a high-incidence country (Japan) to a low-incidence country (Hawaii). According to these surveys, migrants showed the risk rate of their native areas, while their second-generation acquired the risk rate of the host country, thanks to better dietary habits [35]. As a confirmation of this, in Japan, where stomach cancer is still a dominant cancer, a Western-style breakfast showed an inverse association with gastric cancer risk in males [36]. Wheat fiber can neutralize carcinogenic nitrosamines from salivary nitrites [37]. The intake of calcium, vitamin A and C may reduce the N-nitroso compounds concentration [30]. High intakes of fruit and vegetables may reduce the risk by 30–70%; this protective effect seems to be less important for CA [5]. Data on diet can be summarized by the results of a case-control study performed in Uruguay, a country where incidence rates reach high figures. This study confirmed that diets rich in vegetables and fruits and with low amounts of salty (i.e. stewed and processed meat) and starchy foods are recommended for the prevention of gastric cancer [38].

Paralleling esophageal adenocarcinomas, obesity has been considered as another main risk factor for CA in the West, increasing the risk by approximately 50% [19].

Tobacco smoking increases risk of both CA and NCA by two to three times [19,20]. It has been shown that prolonged use of tobacco products is associated with a 1.5 to 2 times increased stomach cancer mortality in men and women [39]. Only a few epidemiologic studies have addressed the role of sex hormones in the etiology of gastric cancer. They have mainly investigated the association with menstrual or reproductive factors, and the results have been contradictory [40,41]. The hypothesis that estrogens may prevent gastric cancer is supported by a nationwide cohort study of men with prostate cancer, that indicated a reduced risk in this cohort exposed to estrogens [42]. Regular, continuing use of NSAIDs was found to be associated with a reduced risk (by about 70%) of stomach cancer [43].

It seems that a number of these factors sometimes play an opposite role in the occurrence of cancers in different gastric subsites, substaining the hypothesis that cardia and proximal gastric cancer be different entities with respect to distal cancers.

Colorectal adenocarcinoma

Colon carcinogenesis results from a loss of genomic stability that leads to the transformation of normal colonic epithelial cells to colon adenocarcinoma cells. Most colorectal cancers arise from benign and asymptomatic colonic polyps, and some factors influencing the risk for colorectal carcinomas (CRC) are responsible for the occurrence of adenomas. Nevertheless, other evidence suggests that many risk factors for colorectal neoplasia may be important to adenoma formation, but not to dysplasia per se [44,45]. It is estimated that 12% of colon cancers are attributable to the following of a Western-style diet, but dietary factors associated with polyp development may not be the same as those associated with cancer [46]. The evidence is consistent for increases in risk associated with animal fat and red meat consumption [47,48]. However, no evidence of a positive association with the frequency of meat consumption was observed among non-vegetarians and vegetarians [49]. In addition, recently The Women's Health Initiative Dietary Modification Trial showed that a low-fat dietary pattern intervention did not reduce the risk of CRC in postmenopausal women [50]. The potential risk-reducing benefits of fruit, vegetable, and fiber consumption for colorectal cancer are less clear [51,52]. The beneficial role of most vegetables was confirmed in an Italian study, which showed a more than 20% reduction in the risk of colorectal cancer from the addition of one daily serving [53]. Among nutrients, beta-carotene, ascorbic acid, folate, selenium, magnesium, calcium are thought to contribute to colon cancer prevention, especially in high risk individuals [54,55], but equivocal evidence exists for dietary antioxidants [56].

The role of alcohol is also controversial. In patients with at least one colorectal adenoma an excessive consumption of alcohol increased the likelihood of developing high risk adenomas or colorectal cancer. A meta-analysis of prospective cohort studies showed a 15% increased risk of colon or rectal cancer for an increase of 100 g of alcohol intake per week. This relationship did not differ significantly by anatomical site [57,58]. On the contrary, no increased risk of colorectal cancer was found among alcoholics by Ye et al. [59].

Several studies strongly support the idea that colorectal cancer might be a tobacco-associated disease, assuming that up to one in five tumors in Western countries may be attributable to tobacco use [49,60]. The major effect of smoking could occur in the earlier stages of the formation of adenomas and of development of carcinoma in situ. Alcohol use, tobacco use, and male gender seem to be associated with earlier onset and a distal location of CRC [61]. The risk for colorectal cancer increases with the length of exposure to smoke, and it may be reduced after long-term smoking cessation [62].

An increased risk for CRC has been associated with obesity and low physical activity, which is inversely associated with the risk of having large polyps.

However, so far the available data are inconsistent [63–65]. Glycemic index has been positively associated with approximately three-fold risk of colorectal cancer. The risk may be mostly explained by glycated hemoglobin concentrations and it is possible that the correlation be due to an indirect role of refined carbohydrates, which are considered general indicators of a poor diet [66,67], but data are contradictory [68,69].

Barrett's esophagus, the main determinant of esophageal adenocarcinoma, has been hypothesized to be an independent risk factor for CRC as well [70]. The protective effect of NSAIDs on CRC was recently questioned by a prospective cohort study from Sturmer *et al.* [71] showing that regular use of these drugs did not succeed in a substantial risk reduction for CRC.

As in the case of gastric cancer, exogenous female hormones are supposed to play a protective role in CRC, too [72]. This could explain in part the decline of mortality rates for the pathology in many developed countries in women, but not in men. Reproductive factors may have differential roles in colon and rectal cancer etiology [73].

Familial history and individual susceptibility

It is proven that some individuals are more prone to develop several pathologies and that an interaction exists between environmental factors and individual susceptibility. It is also possible that in certain cases environmental factors are the main reason for familial clustering of carcinomas and that the expression of familial susceptibility can be modified by adult life risk factors [74].

A positive family history of ESCC or CA has been significantly associated with risk of ESCC and gastric tumors [75], while heredity does not seem to contribute significantly to the occurrence of esophageal cancer according to Lagergren *et al.* [76]. Familial clustering of both BE and EA occurs, but the influence of genetic factors in the etiology of EA is still debated [77]. Gastric cancer can develop as part of the hereditary non-polyposis colon cancer syndrome, as well as part of the gastrointestinal polyposis syndrome, including familial adenomatous polyposis and Peutz–Jeghers syndrome. It has been estimated that approximately 8% of stomach cancers have an inherited familial component [78]. Associations with family history are weakest for rectal cancer and strongest for proximal colonic cancer. Data among spouses and siblings consistently point to the importance of heritable factors in familial CRC: the risks between siblings were increased particularly for cancer in the right-sided colon [79]. According to Negri *et al.* [80] a family history of CRC in first-degree relatives increases the risk of both colon and rectal cancer, the association being stronger at younger ages and for the right colon.

Table 2.6 Studies on genes and gastrointestinal tumors.

	Author	Gene	Results
Esophagus	Cai et al., 2006 [100]	ALDH2, XRCC1	Low dietary selenium and polymorphisms increase the risk of ESCC
	Dandara et al., 2006 [101]	SULT1A1, CYP3A5	The genotype is associated with increased risk for ESCC among smokers
Stomach	Saadat et al., 2006 [102]	GSTM1, GSTT1	Null genotypes increase risk
	Duarte et al., 2005 [103]	XRCC1, XRCC3	Interaction with environmental exposure and risk of chronic gastritis and cancer
Colorectum	Lilla et al., 2006 [104]	NAT1, NAT2	Polymorphisms are associated with tobacco smoke and meat consumption
	Yeh et al., 2005 [105]	XRCC1, XRCC3, XPD	DNA–repair pathways may modulate the risk of CRC

CRC: colorectal cancer; ESCC: esophageal squamous cell carcinoma.

A colonoscopy screening program focusing on first-degree relatives of CRC patients showed that 26% of lesions were hyperplastic polyps, 48% were tubular adenomas, 13% were tubulovillous adenomas, 5% were adenomas with high-grade dysplasia, and 7% were adenocarcinomas [81].

The polymorphism of different genes may simultaneously modulate the risk of the tumors and interact with environmental risk factors. Some metabolic pathways, e.g. those involving folate and heterocyclic amines, may be modified by alterations in relevant genes. Polymorphisms of DNA repair genes, and an imbalance between phase I drug metabolism and phase II detoxification may contribute to the development of these diseases. In addition, the expression of key genes in any of these pathways may be lost by inherited or acquired mutation or by hypermethylation. In Table 2.6 some recent studies on the relation between genes and gastrointestinal tumors are reported.

Conclusions

Carcinomas of the esophagus, stomach, and colorectum are somewhat different entities and multiple factors seem to influence the occurrence of these tumors in males or females and at different ages. However, it is certain that a

Table 2.7 Population attributable risks (%) for some aetiologic factors in gastrointestinal tumors.

Cancer	Author	Attributable risk
Esophageal AC	Engel et al., 2003 [82]	Smoke: 40% High body mass index: 41% Gastroesophageal reflux: 30% Low fruit and vegetable intake: 15%
	Terry et al., 2001 [5]	Fruit and vegetables: <3 servings/ day: 20%
Esophageal squamous cell carcinoma	Engel et al., 2003 [82]	Smoke: 57% Alcohol: 72% Low fruit and vegetable intake: 29%
	Terry et al., 2001 [5]	Fruit and vegetables: <3 servings/ day: 20%
	Negri et al., 1992 [106] for males	Smoking: 71% Elevated alcohol: 45% Low β-carotene: 40%
Cardia AC	Engel et al., 2003 [82]	Smoke: 45% High body mass index: 19%
Distal gastric AC	Engel et al., 2003 [82]	Smoke: 18% History of gastric ulcers: 10% High nitrite intake: 41% *Helicobacter pylori* +: 10%
Gastric AC	Chao et al., 2002 [39] La Vecchia et al., 1995 [107]	Tobacco: 28% men, 14% women Low beta-carotene intake: 48% High traditional foods intake: 40% Low vitamin C intake: 16%
	Sjodahl, 2007 [108] La Vecchia et al., 1992 [78]	Current smoke: 18% Family history: 8%
Colorectal AC	La Vecchia et al., 1996 [109]	Low beta-carotene: 39% Low vitamin C: 14% Low beta-carotene and vitamin C: 43% High red meat intake: 17% High daily meal frequency: 13% Family history of CRC: 4
	La Vecchia et al., 1999 [83]	Low vegetable intake: 22% Low physical activity: 14% High education: 12% Family history of CC: 8%

AC: adenocarcinoma; CC: colon cancer; CRC: colorectal cancer.

large number of these cancers may be preventable by following simple recommendations for improving life quality and that few known risk factors account for the majority of tumors. From a public health viewpoint, the impact of a disease depends on the distribution of exposures in the population and on the strength of the association. Table 2.7 reports some studies on the population attributable risk (PAR) for the study of tumors, i.e. the measure of the proportion of the disease that would have been avoided if all participants were moved to the lowest exposure level with regard the etiologic factors. We can see, for example, that ever smoking, alcohol consumption, and low fruit and vegetable consumption can increase the PAR up to 89% for ESCC, and that ever smoking, high body mass, history of GERD, and low fruit and vegetable consumption account for 79% of EA. Smoking, history of gastric ulcers, high nitrite intake, and *Hp* infection may be responsible for about 59% of distal gastric adenocarcinomas [82]. High education, low physical activity, high energy intake, low vegetable intake, high eating frequency, and a family history of colorectal cancer may account for 56% of colon cancers [83]. In general, lifestyles associated with an increased risk of gastrointestinal tumors are those typical of a diet rich in fat and calories, alcohol, tobacco smoking, and with a low intake of vegetable, fruits, and fibers, and a sedentary lifestyle. Generally speaking, we can say that recommendations for improving lifestyle behavior and the quality of the diet, increasing physical activity, and cessation of smoking are consistent with general recommendations for reducing overall cancer risk.

References

1 Ishii T, Murakami J, Notohara K et al. Oesophageal squamous cell cancer may develop within a background of accumulating DNA methylation in normal and dysplastic mucosa. *Gut* 2006 [Epub ahead of print].
2 Zambon P, Talamini R, La Vecchia C et al. Smoking, type of alcoholic beverage and squamous-cell oesophageal cancer in northern Italy. *Int J Cancer* 2000; **86**: 144–9.
3 Bahmanyar S, Ye W. Dietary patterns and risk of squamous-cell carcinoma and adenocarcinoma of the esophagus and adenocarcinoma of the gastric cardia: a population-based case–control study in Sweden. *Nutr Cancer* 2006; **54**: 171–8.
4 De Stefani E, Boffetta P, Deneo-Pellegrini H et al. The role of vegetable and fruit consumption in the aetiology of squamous cell carcinoma of the oesophagus: a case-control study in Uruguay. *Int J Cancer* 2005; **116**: 130–5.
5 Terry P, Lagergren J, Hansen H et al. Fruit and vegetable consumption in the prevention of oesophageal and cardia cancers. *Eur J Cancer Prev* 2001; **10**: 365–9.
6 Mayne ST, Risch HA, Dubrow R et al. Nutrient intake and risk of subtypes of esophageal and gastric cancer. *Cancer Epidemiol Biomarkers Prev* 2001; **10**: 1055–62.
7 De Stefani E, Deneo-Pellegrini H, Ronco AL et al. Food groups and risk of squamous cell carcinoma of the oesophagus: a case-control study in Uruguay. *Br J Cancer* 2003; **89**: 1209–14.
8 Orengo MA, Casella C, Fontana V et al. Trends in incidence rates of oesophagus and gastric cancer in Italy by subsite and histology, 1986–1997. *Eur J Gastroenterol Hepatol* 2006; **18**: 739–46.
9 Farrow DC, Vaughan TL, Sweeney C et al. Gastroesophageal reflux disease, use of H2 receptor antagonists, and risk of esophageal and gastric cancer. *Cancer Causes Control* 2000; **11**: 231–8.
10 Wu AH, Tseng CC, Bernstein L. Hiatal hernia, reflux symptoms, body size, and risk of esophageal and gastric adenocarcinoma. *Cancer* 2003; **98**: 940–8.
11 De Jonge PJ, Steyerberg EW, Kuipers et al. Risk factors for the development of esophageal adenocarcinoma in Barrett's esophagus. *Am J Gastroenterol* 2006; **101**: 1421–9.
12 Conio M, Blanchi S, Lapertosa G et al. Long-term endoscopic surveillance of patients with Barrett's esophagus. Incidence of dysplasia and adenocarcinoma: a prospective study. *Am J Gastroenterol* 2003; **98**: 1931–9.

13 Spechler SJ, Robbins AH, Rubins HB *et al*. Adenocarcinoma and Barrett's esophagus. An over-rated risk? *Gastroenterology* 1984; **87**: 927–33.

14 Ronkainen J Aro P, Storskrubb T *et al*. Prevalence of Barrett's esophagus in the general population: an endoscopic study. *Gastroenterology* 2005; **129**: 1825–31.

15 Weston AP, Badr AS, Topalovski M *et al*. Prospective evaluation of the prevalence of gastric Helicobacter pylori infection in patients with GERD, Barrett's esophagus, Barrett's dysplasia, and Barrett's adenocarcinoma. *Am J Gastroenterol* 2000; **95**: 387–94.

16 Ye W , Held M, Lagergren J *et al*. Helicobacter pylori infection and gastric atrophy: risk of adenocarcinoma and squamous-cell carcinoma of the esophagus and gastric cardia adenocarcinoma. *J Natl Cancer Inst* 2004; **96**: 388–96.

17 Wu AH, Crabtree JE, Bernstein L *et al*. Role of Helicobacter pylori CagA+ strains and risk of adenocarcinoma of the stomach and esophagus. *Int J Cancer* 2003; **103**: 815–21.

18 Terry P, Lagergren J, Ye W *et al*. Antioxidants and cancers of the esophagus and gastric cardia. *Int J Cancer* 2000; **87**: 750–4.

19 Lindblad M, Rodriguez LA, Lagergren J. Body mass, tobacco and alcohol and risk of esophageal, gastric cardia, and gastric non-cardia adenocarcinoma among men and women in a nested case-control study. *Cancer Causes Control* 2005; **16**: 285–94.

20 Wu AH, Wan P, Bernstein L. A multiethnic population-based study of smoking, alcohol and body size and risk of adenocarcinomas of the stomach and esophagus (United States). *Cancer Causes Control* 2001; **12**: 721–32.

21 Lagergren J. Controversies surrounding body mass, reflux, and risk of oesophageal adenocarcinoma. *Lancet Oncology* 2006; **7**: 347–9.

22 Avidan B, Sonnenberg A, Schnell TG *et al*. Hiatal hernia size, Barrett's length, and severity of acid reflux are all risk factors for esophageal adenocarcinoma. *Am J Gastroenterol* 2002; **97**: 1930–6.

23 Gammon MD, Schoenberg JB, Ahsan H *et al*. Tobacco, alcohol, and socioeconomic status and adenocarcinoma of the esophagus and gastric cardia. *J Natl Cancer Inst* 1997; **89**: 1277–84.

24 Levi F, Ollyo JB, Vecchia C *et al*. The consumption of tobacco, alcohol and the risk of adeno-carcinoma in Barrett's esophagus. *Int J Cancer* 1990; **15**: 852–4.

25 Souza RF, Shewmake K, Beer DG *et al*. Selective inhibition of cyclooxygenase-2 suppresses growth and induces apoptosis in human esophageal adenocarcinoma cells. *Cancer Res* 2000; **60**: 5767–72.

26 Lynch HT, Grady W, Suriano G *et al*. Gastric cancer: new genetic developments. *J Surg Oncol* 2005; **90**: 114–33.

27 Bernini M, Barbi S, Roviello F *et al*. Family history of gastric cancer: a correlation between epidemiologic findings and clinical data. *Gastric Cancer* 2006; **9**: 9–13.

28 Weck MN, Brenner H. Prevalence of chronic atrophic gastritis in different parts of the world. *Cancer Epidemiol Biomarkers Prev* 2006; **15**: 1083–94.

29 Borch K, Jonsson KA, Petersson F *et al*. Prevalence of gastroduodenitis and Helicobacter pylori infection in a general population sample: relations to symptomatology and life-style. *Dig Dis Sci* 2000; **45**: 1322–9.

30 Dicken BJ, Bigam DL, Cass C *et al*. Gastric adenocarcinoma: review and considerations for future directions. *Ann Surg* 2005; **241**: 27–39.

31 Gonzalez CA, Jakszyn P, Pera G *et al*. Meat intake and risk of stomach and esophageal adeno-carcinoma within the European Prospective Investigation Into Cancer and Nutrition (EPIC). *J Natl Cancer Inst* 2006; **98**: 345–54.

32 Parsonnet J, Friedman GD, Vandersteen DP *et al*. Helicobacter pylori infection and the risk of gastric carcinoma. *N Engl J Med* 1991; **325**: 1127–31.

33 Knekt P, Teppo L, Aromaa A *et al*. Helicobacter pylori IgA and IgG antibodies, serum pepsinogen I and the risk of gastric cancer: changes in the risk with extended follow-up period. *Int J Cancer* 2006; **119**: 702–5.

34 Kamangar F, Dawsey SM, Blaser MJ *et al*. Opposing risks of gastric cardia and noncardia gastric adenocarcinomas associated with Helicobacter pylori seropositivity. *J Natl Cancer Inst* 2006; **98**: 1445–52.

35 Haenszel W, Kurihara M. Studies of Japanese migrants. I. Mortality from cancer and other diseases among Japanese in the United States. *J Natl Cancer Inst* 1968; **40**: 43–68.

36 Tokui N, Yoshimura T, Fujino Y *et al*. Dietary habits and stomach cancer risk in the JACC Study. *J Epidemiol* 2005; **15**: S98–S108.

37 Nomura AM, Hankin JH, Kolonel LN *et al*. Case-control study of diet and other risk factors for gastric cancer in Hawaii (United States). *Cancer Causes Control* 2003; **14**: 547–58.

38 De Stefani E, Correa P, Boffetta P *et al*. Dietary patterns and risk of gastric cancer: a case-control study in Uruguay. *Gastric Cancer* 2004; **7**: 211–20.

39 Chao A, Thun MJ, S. Henley J *et al*. Cigarette smoking, use of other tobacco products and stomach cancer mortality in US adults: The cancer Prevention Study II. *Int J Cancer* 2002; **101**: 380–9.

40 Heuch I, Kvale G. Menstrual and reproductive factors and risk of gastric cancer: a Norwegian cohort study. *Cancer Causes Control* 2000; **11**: 869–74.

41 La Vecchia C, D'Avanzo B, Franceschi S *et al*. Menstrual and reproductive factors and gastric-cancer risk in women. *Int J Cancer* 1994; **59**: 761–4.

42. Lindblad M, Ye W, Rubio C *et al*. Estrogen and risk of gastric cancer: a protective effect in a nationwide cohort study of patients with prostate cancer in Sweden. *Cancer Epidemiol Biomarkers Prev* 2004; **13**: 2203–7.

43 Coogan PF, Rosenberg L, Palmer JR *et al*. Nonsteroidal anti-inflammatory drugs and risk of digestive cancers at sites other than the large bowel. *Cancer Epidemiol Biomarkers Prev* 2000; **9**: 119–23.

44 Terry MB, Neugut AI, Bostick RM *et al*. Risk factors for advanced colorectal adenomas: a pooled analysis. *Cancer Epidemiol Biomarkers Prev* 2002; **11**(7): 622–9.

45 Breuer-Katschinski B, Nemes K, Marr A *et al*. Alcohol and cigarette smoking and the risk of colorectal adenomas. *Dig Dis Sci* 2000; **45**: 487–93.

46 Yoon H, Benamouzig R, Little J *et al*. Systematic review of epidemiological studies on meat, dairy products and egg consumption and risk of colorectal adenomas. *Eur J Cancer Prev* 2000; **9**: 151–64.

47 Larsson SC, Rafter J, Holmberg L *et al*. Red meat consumption and risk of cancers of the proximal colon, distal colon and rectum: the Swedish Mammography Cohort. *Int J Cancer* 2005; **113**: 829–34.

48 Norat T, Bingham S, Ferrari P *et al*. Meat, fish, and colorectal cancer risk: the European Prospective Investigation into cancer and nutrition. *J Natl Cancer Inst* 2005; **97**: 906–16.

49 Sanjoaquin MA, Appleby PN, Thorogood M *et al*. Nutrition, lifestyle and colorectal cancer incidence: a prospective investigation of 10 998 vegetarians and non-vegetarians in the United Kingdom. *Br J Cancer* 2004; **90**: 118–21.

50 Beresford SA, Johnson KC, Ritenbaugh C *et al*. Low-fat dietary pattern and risk of colorectal cancer: the Women's Health Initiative Randomized Controlled Dietary Modification Trial. *JAMA* 2006; **295**: 643–54.

51 Lin J, Zhang SM, Cook NR *et al*. Dietary intakes of fruit, vegetables, and fiber, and risk of colorectal cancer in a prospective cohort of women (United States). *Cancer Causes Control* 2005; **16**: 225–33.

52 Peters U, Sinha R, Chatterjee N *et al*. Dietary fibre and colorectal adenoma in a colorectal cancer early detection programme. *Lancet* 2003; **361**: 1491–5.

53 Franceschi S, Favero A, La Vecchia C *et al*. Food groups and risk of colorectal cancer in Italy. *Int J Cancer* 1997; **72**: 56–61.

54 Folsom AR, Hong CP. Magnesium intake and reduced risk of colon cancer in a prospective study of women. *Am J Epidemiol* 2006; **163**: 232.

55 Larsson SC, Bergkvist L, Rutegard J *et al*. Calcium and dairy food intakes are inversely associated with colorectal cancer risk in the Cohort of Swedish Men. *Am J Clin Nutr* 2006; **83**: 667–73.

56 Malila N, Virtamo J, Virtanen M *et al*. Dietary and serum alpha-tocopherol, beta-carotene and retinol, and risk for colorectal cancer in male smokers. *Eur J Clin Nutr* 2002; **56**: 615–21.

57 Cho E, Smith-Warner SA, Ritz J *et al*. Alcohol intake and colorectal cancer: a pooled analysis of 8 cohort studies. *Ann Intern Med* 2004; **140**: 603–13.

58 Moskal A, Norat T, Ferrari P *et al*. Alcohol intake and colorectal cancer risk: a dose-response meta-analysis of published cohort studies. *Int J Cancer* 2007; **120**: 664–71.

59 Ye W, Romelsjo A, Augustsson K *et al*. No excess risk of colorectal cancer among alcoholics followed for up to 25 years. *Br J Cancer* 2003; **88**: 1044–6.

60 Giovannucci E. An updated review of the epidemiological evidence that cigarette smoking increases risk of colorectal cancer. *Cancer Epidemiol Biomarkers Prev* 2001; **10**: 725–31.

61 Zisman AL, Nickolov A, Brand RE *et al*. Associations between the age at diagnosis and location of colorectal cancer and the use of alcohol and tobacco: implications for screening. *Arch Intern Med* 2006; **166**: 629–34.

62 Verla-Tebit E, Lilla C, Hoffmeister M *et al*. Cigarette smoking and colorectal cancer risk in Germany: a population-based case-control study. *Int J Cancer* 2006; **119**: 630–5.

63 Engeland A, Tretli S, Austad G *et al*. Height and body mass index in relation to colorectal and gallbladder cancer in two million Norwegian men and women. *Cancer Causes Control* 2005; **16**: 987–96.

64 Pischon T, Lahmann PH, Boeing H *et al*. Body size and risk of colon and rectal cancer in the European Prospective Investigation into Cancer and Nutrition (EPIC). *J Natl Cancer Inst* 2006; **98**: 920–31.

65 Larsson SC, Rutegard J, Bergkvist L *et al*. Physical activity, obesity, and risk of colon and rectal cancer in a cohort of Swedish men. *Eur J Cancer* 2006; **42**: 2590–7.

66 Khaw KT, Wareham N, Bingham S *et al*. Preliminary communication: glycated hemoglobin, diabetes, and incident colorectal cancer in men and women: a prospective analysis from the European prospective investigation into cancer – Norfolk study. *Cancer Epidemiol Biomarkers Prev* 2004; **13**: 915–19.

67 Limburg PJ, Vierkant RA, Fredericksen ZS *et al*. Clinically confirmed type 2 diabetes mellitus and colorectal cancer risk: a population-based, retrospective cohort study. *Am J Gastroenterol* 2006; **101**: 1872–9.

68 Oh K, Willett WC, Fuchs CS *et al*. Glycemic index, glycemic load, and carbohydrate intake in relation to risk of distal colorectal adenoma in women. *Cancer Epidemiol Biomarkers Prev* 2004; **13**: 1192–8.

69 McCarl M, Harnack L, Limburg PJ *et al*. Incidence of colorectal cancer in relation to glycemic index and load in a cohort of women. *Cancer Epidemiol Biomarkers Prev* 2006; **15**: 892–6.

70 Siersema PD, Yu S, Sahbaie P *et al*. Colorectal neoplasia in veterans is associated with Barrett's esophagus but not with proton-pump inhibitor or aspirin/NSAID use. *Gastrointest Endosc* 2006; **63**: 581–6.

71 Sturmer T, Buring JE, Lee IM *et al*. Colorectal cancer after start of nonsteroidal antiinflammatory drug use. *Am J Med* 2006; **119**: 494–502.

72 Fernandez E, Gallus S, Bosetti C *et al*. Hormone replacement therapy and cancer risk: a systematic analysis from a network of case-control studies. *Int J Cancer* 2003; **105**: 408–12.

73 Nichols HB, Trentham-Dietz A, Hampton JM *et al*. Oral contraceptive use, reproductive factors, and colorectal cancer risk: findings from Wisconsin. *Cancer Epidemiol Biomarkers Prev* 2005; **14**: 1212–18.

74 Fernandez E, Gallus S, La Vecchia C *et al*. Family history and environmental risk factors for colon cancer. *Cancer Epidemiol Biomarkers Prev* 2004; **13**: 658–61.

75 Tran GD, Sun XD, Abnet CC *et al*. Prospective study of risk factors for esophageal and gastric cancers in the Linxian general population trial cohort in China. *Int J Cancer* 2005; **113**(3): 456–63.

76 Lagergren J, Ye W, Lindgren A *et al*. Heredity and risk of cancer of the esophagus and gastric cardia. *Cancer Epidemiol Biomarkers Prev* 2000; **9**: 757–60.

77 Chak A, Lee T, Kinnard MF *et al*. Familial aggregation of Barrett's oesophagus, oesophageal adenocarcinoma, and oesophagogastric junctional adenocarcinoma in Caucasian adults. *Gut* 2002; **51**: 323–8.

78 La Vecchia C, Negri E, Franceschi S *et al*. Family history and the risk of stomach and colorectal cancer. *Cancer* 1992; **70**: 50–5.

79 Hemminki K, Chen B. Familial risk for colorectal cancers are mainly due to heritable causes. *Cancer Epidemiol Biomarkers Prev* 2004; **13**: 1253–6.

80 Negri E, Braga C, La Vecchia C *et al*. Family history of cancer and risk of colorectal cancer in Italy. *Br J Cancer* 1998; **77**: 174–9.

81 Pezzoli A, Matarese V, Rubini M *et al*. Colorectal cancer screening: results of a 5-year program in asymptomatic subjects at increased risk. *Dig Liver Dis* 2006 [Epub ahead of print].

82 Engel LS, Chow WH, Vaughan TL *et al*. Population attributable risks of esophageal and gastric cancers. *J Natl Cancer Inst* 2003; **95**: 1404–13.

83 La Vecchia C, Braga C, Franceschi S, *et al*. Population-attributable risk for colon cancer in Italy. *Nutr Cancer* 1999; **33**: 196–200.

84 Gallus S, Altieri A, Bosetti C *et al*. Cigarette tar yield and risk of upper digestive tract cancers: case-control studies from Italy and Switzerland. *Ann Oncol* 2003; **14**: 209–13.

85 Sasazuki S, Sasaki S, Tsugane S. Japan Public Health Center Study Group. Cigarette smoking, alcohol consumption and subsequent gastric cancer risk by subsite and histologic type. *Int J Cancer* 2002; **101**: 560–6.

86 Fujino Y, Mizoue T, Tokui N *et al*. Cigarette smoking and mortality due to stomach cancer: findings from the JACC Study. *J Epidemiol* 2005; **15**: S13–19.

87 Limburg PJ, Vierkant RA, Cerhan JR *et al*. Cigarette smoking and colorectal cancer: long-term, subsite-specific risks in a cohort study of postmenopausal women. *Clin Gastroenterol Hepatol* 2003; **1**: 202–10.

88 Engeland A, Tretli S, Bjorge T. Height and body mass index in relation to esophageal cancer; 23-year follow-up of two million Norwegian men and women. *Cancer Causes Control* 2004; **15**: 837–43.

89 Vigen C, Bernstein L, Wu AH. Occupational physical activity and risk of adenocarcinomas of the esophagus and stomach. *Int J Cancer* 2006; **118**: 1004–9.

90 Kubo A, Corley DA. Body mass index and adenocarcinomas of the esophagus or gastric cardia: a systematic review and meta-analysis. *Cancer Epidemiol Biomarkers Prev* 2006; **15**: 872–8.

91 Lin J, Zhang SM, Cook NR *et al*. Body mass index and risk of colorectal cancer in women (United States). *Cancer Causes Control* 2004; **15**: 581–9.

92 Franceschi S, Dal Maso L, Augustin L *et al*. Dietary glycemic load and colorectal cancer risk. *Ann Oncol* 2001; **12**:173–8.

93 Mao Y, Pan S, Wen SW *et al*. Physical inactivity, energy intake, obesity and the risk of rectal cancer in Canada. *Int J Cancer* 2003; **105**: 831–7.

94 Bollschweiler E, Wolfgarten E, Nowroth T *et al*. Vitamin intake and risk of subtypes of esophageal cancer in Germany. *J Cancer Res Clin Oncol* 2002; **128**: 575–80.

95 Kobayashi M, Tsubono Y, Sasazuki S *et al*. Vegetables, fruit and risk of gastric cancer in Japan: a 10-year follow-up of the JPHC Study Cohort I. *Int J Cancer* 2002; **102**(1): 39–44.

96 Larsson SC, Bergkvist L, Wolk A. Processed meat consumption, dietary nitrosamines and stomach cancer risk in a cohort of Swedish women. *Int J Cancer* 2006; **119**(4): 915–19.

97 Lin J, Zhang SM, Cook NR. Dietary intakes of fruit, vegetables, and fiber, and risk of colorectal cancer in a prospective cohort of women (United States). *Cancer Causes Control* 2005; **16**: 225–33.

98 Larsson SC, Giovannucci E, Wolk A. A prospective study of dietary folate intake and risk of colorectal cancer: modification by caffeine intake and cigarette smoking. *Cancer Epidemiol Biomarkers Prev* 2005; **14**: 740–3.

99 Larsson SC, Wolk A. Meat consumption and risk of colorectal cancer: a meta-analysis of prospective studies. *Int J Cancer* 2006; **119**: 2657–64.

100 Cai L, You NC, Lu H *et al*. Dietary selenium intake, aldehyde dehydrogenase-2 and X-ray repair cross-complementing 1 genetic polymorphisms, and the risk of esophageal squamous cell carcinoma. *Cancer* 2006; **106**: 2345–54.

101 Dandara C, Li DP, Walther G *et al*. Gene-environment interaction: the role of SULT1A1 and CYP3A5 polymorphisms as risk modifiers for squamous cell carcinoma of the oesophagus. *Carcinogenesis* 2006; **274**: 91–7.

102 Saadat M. Genetic polymorphisms of glutathione S-transferase T1 (GSTT1) and susceptibility to gastric cancer: a meta-analysis. *Cancer Sci* 2006; **97**: 505–9.

103 Duarte MC, Colombo J, Rossit AR *et al.* Polymorphisms of DNA repair genes XRCC1 and XRCC3, interaction with environmental exposure and risk of chronic gastritis and gastric cancer. *World J Gastroenterol* 2005; **11**(42): 6593–600.

104 Lilla C, Verla-Tebit E, Risch A *et al.* Effect of NAT1 and NAT2 genetic polymorphisms on colorectal cancer risk associated with exposure to tobacco smoke and meat consumption. *Cancer Epidemiol Biomarkers Prev* 2006; **15**: 99–107.

105 Yeh CC, Sung FC, Tang R *et al.* Polymorphisms of the XRCC1, XRCC3, & XPD genes, and colorectal cancer risk: a case-control study in Taiwan. *BMC* 2005; 5:12.

106 Negri E, La Vecchia C, Franceschi S *et al.* Attributable risks for oesophageal cancer in Northern Italy. *Eur J Cancer* 1992; **28**: 1167–71.

107 La Vecchia C, D'Avanzo B, Negri E *et al.* Attributable risks for stomach cancer in northern Italy. *Int J Cancer* 1995; **60**: 748–52.

108 Sjodahl K, Lu Y, Nilsen TI *et al.* Smoking and alcohol drinking in relation to risk of gastric cancer: a population-based, prospective cohort study. *Int J Cancer* 2007; **120**: 128–32.

109 La Vecchia C, Ferraroni M, Mezzetti M *et al.* Attributable risks for colorectal cancer in northern Italy. *Int J Cancer* 1996; **66**: 60–4.

CHAPTER 3

Staging before EMR

PETER D. SIERSEMA AND PAUL FOCKENS

Introduction

Historically, the detection of high-grade intra-epithelial neoplasia (HGIN) and early-stage cancer in the gastrointestinal (GI) tract, i.e. intramucosal (T1m) or submucosal (T1sm) cancer, is mostly performed with videoendoscopy, which is able to detect gross mucosal lesions in the GI tract, such as elevations, ulcerations, and nodularity. More careful and thorough inspection is however needed to detect early lesions.

Detection of these abnormalities has been improved by the development of new endoscopic modalities, particularly with regard to: (a) white light endoscopy, particularly high-resolution endoscopy (HRE), high magnification endoscopy and chromoendoscopy; (b) optical spectroscopy; and (c) endomicroscopy, represented by endocystoscopy and laser confocal microscopy. The pros and cons and results of these techniques in detecting early neoplastic lesions in the GI tract are discussed in Chapter 4: Advances in Endoscopic Imaging of Barrett's Esophagus.

Although some of these new modalities play a role in staging early neoplastic lesions, the mainstay in the staging process is endoscopic ultrasound (EUS). In this chapter we will discuss the available staging modalities for early cancer of the esophagus, stomach, and colorectum.

Esophagus

The endoscopic diagnosis and staging of esophageal carcinoma is relatively straightforward since patients usually are diagnosed with advanced tumors that are easily recognizable by endoscopy. The true challenge is the detection of early neoplastic lesions of the esophagus. If these lesions are histologically confirmed, the next step is staging with the aim of determining whether an endoscopic resection is feasible.

Endoscopic Mucosal Resection. Edited by M. Conio, P. Siersema, A. Repici and T. Ponchon. © 2008 Blackwell Publishing. ISBN 978-1-4051-5885-5.

High-resolution endoscopy

In the last two decades, endoscopes with charge-coupled devices (CCD), i.e. electronic endoscopes, have largely replaced fibreoptic endoscopes. The CCDs in a standard videoendoscope used to contain hundred 38000–300 000 pixels. Recently, endoscopes containing CCDs with 600 000 to 1 million pixels have been introduced. These are called high-resolution endoscopes (HRE). High resolution now seem to have become the new standard for endoscopic imaging.

May *et al.* [1] performed a study in which HRE was used to stage patients with early esophageal adenocarcinoma (*n*=81) or squamous cell carcinoma (*n*=19). Polypoid, depressed, and excavated configurations and ulcerations were regarded as endoscopic signs with a higher risk of submucosal infiltration. Results were correlated with the histological result obtained by endoscopic mucosal resection (EMR). Overall accuracy of staging with HRE was 83%. Sensitivity for mucosal (T1m) tumors was higher than 94%, while that for submucosal (T1sm) tumors was only 56%.

Endoscopic ultrasound

Anatomy of the normal esophageal wall
The GI tract wall comprises four distinct histologic layers, i.e. the mucosa, submucosa, muscularis propria, and adventitia (Fig. 3.1). The innermost layer is the superficial mucosa and is represented as a hyperechoic band by EUS. In reality, this layer represents the initial echo-interface between the ultrasound waves, the GI tract mucosa, and the surrounding fluid. The second hypoechoic layer represents the deep mucosa, including the muscularis mucosae. The third hyperechoic layer corresponds histologically with the submucosa. The fourth hypoechoic layer represents the muscularis propria, whereas the fifth hyperechoic layer is the adventitial layer. The normal esophageal wall measures 3–4 mm in the distal esophagus. Areas of focal thickening are suspicious for the presence of carcinoma.

Distinguishing between T1m and T1sm early esophageal cancer
It should be noted that the risk of lymph node metastases increases rapidly with tumors invading the esophageal submucosa (T1sm) [2]. T1m squamous cell carcinomas have a less than 4% risk of lymph node metastases, but this risk is more than 25% for T1sm tumors. This is also true for adenocarcinomas, with lymph node metastases in 2% of T1m and 27% of T1sm tumors [3].

EMR is an attractive alternative to esophagectomy, particularly for T1m esophageal cancers, as the risk of dying from metastatic disease (varying between

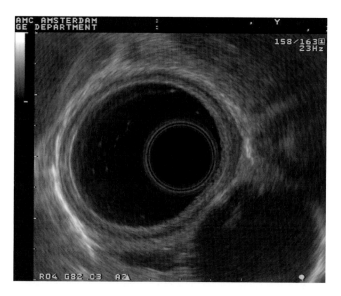

Fig. 3.1 The wall of a normal esophagus comprising four distinct histologic layers, i.e. the mucosa, submucosa, muscularis propria, and adventitia.

1.9% and 3.7%) in this situation is lower than that of a surgical procedure. It is known that the mortality due to esophagectomy varies between 3% and 5%, with significant morbidity in 30% of cases, even in expert centers [4].

In addition, EMR is able to give prognostic information, as it allows histological examination of the resected specimen with regard to the depth of infiltration (involvement of the mucosa (T1m) and submucosa (T1sm)), extension of the tumor into the base and lateral margins, degree of infiltration, and, in some cases, invasion of lymphatic vessels and veins. This information is however only available after an EMR has already been performed.

Staging before EMR is clinically important for defining the subgroup of patients that are most likely to be good candidates for an endoscopic therapeutic option. On the other hand, if the histological examination of the EMR specimen shows that the lesion is extending into the submucosa, a surgical resection is still possible. Therefore, EMR can also be considered to be a diagnostic procedure in these situations. Other imaging methods such as EUS are in that case only used to exclude metastatic disease (N or M).

EUS method

In general, high-frequency (20–30 MHz) probes are used to determine tumor infiltration into the different layers of the wall of the GI tract, whereas low-frequency (7.5–12.5 MHz) probes are used to detect the presence of metastases in lymph nodes or other organs such as the liver.

The main advantage of evaluating the esophagus with high-frequency EUS probes is the higher resolution of images compared to low-frequency probes. With these high-frequency miniprobes, it is possible to discriminate nine different layers. In this nine-layer concept the first four layers are all mucosal with the fourth layer representing the muscularis mucosae. The miniprobes are 2–3 mm in diameter and can be passed through the working channel of a standard or therapeutic endoscope.

Enlarged peri-esophageal, celiac, and posterior mediastinal lymph nodes are easily detected with EUS. Lymph nodes generally appear darker ('hypoechoic') than surrounding fat or soft tissues (Fig. 3.2). Ultrasonographic features suggestive of malignancy include a round (vs. any other) shape, sharply demarcated borders, hypoechogenicity, and an enlarged size (>5–10 mm) [5].

EUS is increasingly combined with fine-needle aspiration (FNA) to confirm metastatic disease in lymph nodes, particularly if the FNA result will affect a clinical decision [6]. Care should be taken not to perform an EUS–FNA procedure through an esophageal tumor because this may lead to false positive results.

Findings at EUS
Various studies have reported on T and N staging of early esophageal cancer [1,7–12).

T stage.   From these studies, it can be concluded that the combined sensitivity of T1 staging is 80% (Table 3.1). Only one small study, including nine patients,

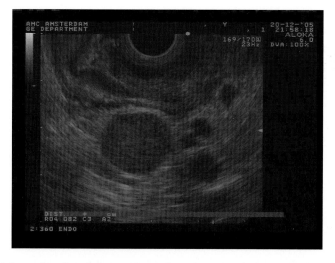

Fig. 3.2 Malignant lymph node (center) in esophageal cancer, which is darker ('hypoechoic') than surrounding fat or soft tissues.

Table 3.1 Reported endoscopic ultrasound (EUS) results on T1 staging in patients with high-grade intra-epithelial neoplasia (HGIN) or early esophageal cancer (EC).

Author	N	Biopsy result (n)	Probe (MHz)	Sensitivity T1 (%)	Specificity T1 (%)	Sensitivity T1m (%)	Specificity T1m (%)	PPV T1m (%)	NPV T1m (%)	Sensitivity T1sm (%)	Specificity T1sm (%)	PPV T1sm (%)	NPV T1sm (%)
Scotiniotis et al. [7]	22	HGIN (10) EC (12)	7.5/12							5/5 (100)	16/17 (94)		16/16 (100)
May et al. [1]	94	EC (94)	20	75/94 (80) (Acc.: 74/93 (83))		62/68 (91)				12/25 (48)			
Buskens et al. [8]	77	HGIN (13) EC (64)	12/20/30							20/21 (95)	19/24 (79)	20/25 (80)	19/20 (95)
Larghi et al. [9]	48	HGIN (25) EC (23)	5–20	41/48 (85)		34/40 (85)				7/8 (88)			
Waxman et al. [10]	9	HGIN (7) EC (2)	5/12	1/3 (33)	3/4 (75)								
Pech et al. [11]	100	EC (100)	7.5 + 12.5/20	42/55 (76) (Acc.: 42/55 (76))		39/44 (89)	3/11 (27)	39/47 (83)	3/8 (38)	3/11 (27)	39/44 (89)	3/8 (38)	39/47 (83)
Shimoyama et al. [12]	20	EC (20)	7.5 + 12–20			Acc.: T1m1–2/m3–sm1/sm2–3: 70%				12/14 (86)			
Total	370	HGIN (55) EC (315)		159/200 (80)	3/4 (75)	135/152 (89)	3/11 (27)	39/47 (83)	3/8 (38)	59/84 (70)	74/85 (87)	23/33 (70)	74/83 (89)

NPV: negative predictive value; PPV: positive predictive value.

gave results on specificity of T1 tumors, which was 75% (3/4) [10]. The combined sensitivity of T1m tumors was 89%, while that of T1sm tumors was lower, at 70% (Table 3.1). One study reported the specificity of T1m tumors, which was only 27% in that study [11]. In contrast, the combined specificity of T1sm tumors was 87%. This translated into a high positive predictive value (PPV) of EUS for T1m tumors and a high negative predictive value (NPV) for T1sm tumors, at 83% and 89%, respectively.

The results show that, when EUS is inaccurate, it tends to overstage rather than to understage. This will result in a decision to perform an esophageal resection in these patients, which is in fact not desirable as an EMR would have been sufficient in the majority of these people. Since understaging rarely occurs, very few patients will be treated with an EMR when the preferred approach would have been a surgical resection. In the latter situation, EMR can however be considered to be a diagnostic procedure, which can still be followed by a more invasive (surgical) procedure. The low morbidity and absent mortality add to the use of EMR as a diagnostic method in experienced hands.

N stage.   For N staging in early esophageal cancer, EUS is considered to be most important, as the finding of positive peri-esophageal, celiac, and posterior mediastinal lymph nodes means that EMR is no longer indicated, and a surgical resection with or without neoadjuvant chemoradiotherapy is the only treatment option. Cytological proof through EUS–FNA is mandatory.

If the results of the four studies that reported on N staging are taken together (Table 3.2), sensitivities varied between 43% and 100%, whereas results for specificity were less different, varying between 71% and 97%. An issue in these studies is however that it is more difficult to define the gold standard as compared to studies in which T stage is evaluated. In three of four studies, the gold standard was the surgical specimen, whereas in another study the gold standard was follow-up by EUS and CT at 6-month intervals [11].

Computed tomography

A major part of the standardized staging procedure in esophageal cancer is thoracic and abdominal computed tomography (CT) to detect the presence of metastatic disease. EUS has been demonstrated to be superior to CT for T and N staging in patients with esophageal cancer [13]. Pech *et al.* [11] compared CT chest/abdomen with high-frequency EUS in 100 patients with T1 esophageal cancer. However, CT had no influence on TNM stage in any of these patients.

Table 3.2 Reported endoscopic ultrasound (EUS) results on N staging in patients with high-grade intra-epithelial neoplasia (HGIN) or early esophageal cancer (EC).

Author	N	Biopsy result (n)	Probe (MHz)	Sensitivity N stage (%)	Specificity N stage (%)	PPV N stage (%)	NPV N stage (%)
Scotiniotis et al. [7]	22	HGD (10) EC (12)	7.5/12	1/1 (100)	17/21 (81)		17/17 (100)
Buskens et al. [8]	77	HGD (13) EC (64)	12/20/30	8/14 (57)	57/61 (94)	8/14 (57)	57/61 (93)
Pech et al. [11]	100	EC (100)	7.5 + 12.5/20	75%	97%	75%	98%
Shimoyama et al. [12]	20	EC (20)	7.5 + 12–20	43% (Acc.: 57%)	71%	60%	56%

HGD: high-grade dysplasia; NPV: negative predictive value; PPV: positive predictive value.

Conclusion

EUS with high- (12–30 MHz) and low- (7.5 MHz) frequency EUS probes is the investigation of choice in patients with early (T1) esophageal cancer to detect more deeply invading tumors and/or metastatic lymph nodes, which would preclude the use of EMR. An endoscopic treatment should mainly be offered if neoplasia is limited to mucosal (T1m1–3) and selected submucosal (T1sm1) tumors without malignant-appearing or demonstrated (by FNA) lymph nodes. There is no additional role for HRE in the staging of these early lesions, whereas a CT should be reserved for patients with more advanced esophageal tumors to detect (distant) metastases.

Stomach

Early gastric cancer is detected by careful endoscopic examination of the stomach and is histologically confirmed by biopsy. For detecting early stage gastric cancer, it is important to realize that subtle changes in color and mucosal pattern may be indicative of an early lesion. It is generally considered to be difficult to diagnose early neoplastic changes in the stomach, at least for Western endoscopists. If an early gastric cancer is found, however, the next step is to determine whether the lesion can be removed by endoscopic means or should be treated with a (partial) gastrectomy.

Videoendoscopy

It would be of clinical value if standard videoendoscopy could predict whether a small gastric lesion, which is suspected to be malignant, is still limited to the mucosa or is already extending into the submucosa of the gastric wall.

Yanai *et al.* [14] compared staging characteristics of endoscopy, using an Olympus GIF-2T200 endoscope with 100 000–300 000 pixels, and conventional EUS in 59 patients with suspected early gastric cancer, and compared these with the gold standard, an endoscopically or surgically resected specimen. Lesions that protruded from the mucosa with a smooth surface and those with a shallow and smooth surfaced depression were classified as mucosal (endoscopy-mucosal). Lesions considered to exhibit submucosal invasion (endoscopy-submucosal) were those that showed a more uneven base, with an irregularly shaped nodule, or those with folds that were enlarged. Overall accuracy rate in staging invasion depth was similar, i.e. 63% for endoscopy and 71% for EUS. Both endoscopy and EUS tended to overstage lesions, in 46% and 43% of patients, respectively, showing submucosal lesions, which were histologically demonstrated to be mucosal. The errors of endoscopy mainly resulted from inadequate interpretation of the depth of the depression, unevenness of the surface, and ulcerous changes.

Magnification endoscopy

Magnification endoscopy in the stomach is often performed in combination with installation of acetic acid [15,16]. Although five different types of surface patterns could be discriminated, no correlation was found between depth of invasivion (mucosa vs. submucosa vs. deeper invasion) and surface pattern. On the other hand, magnification endoscopy was able to determine the extent of horizontal spread of gastric lesions.

Endoscopic ultrasound

Anatomy of the normal gastric wall
On EUS, the normal gastric wall is not different from that of the normal esophagus and is also visualized as having a five-layer architecture. In the stomach, the 5th hyperechoic layer represents the serosa, including the subserosa, and not the adventitia as in the esophagus. Using a high-frequency EUS probe, the fine hypoechoic layer (about 0.2 mm in thickness) between the 2nd and the 3rd hyperechoic layers, which is considered to be the muscularis mucosae, gives information on the depth of invasion of tumors.

Distinguishing between T1m and T1sm early gastric cancer
Similar to the esophagus, the risk of lymph node metastases increases rapidly with tumors invading the gastric submucosa (T1sm). Although the risk of lymph node metastases is low for mucosal lesions, varying between 1.9% and 3.5%, it increases to 14–27% for tumors invading the submucosa [17]. This means that T1m gastric tumors can be considered to be removable by EMR, while a T1sm tumor should be considered to be an indication for partial or total gastrectomy.

EUS method
In general, high-frequency (20–30 MHz) EUS probes are also used in the stomach to determine tumor infiltration into the different layers of the wall of the GI tract, whereas low-frequency (7.5–12.5 MHz) probes are used to detect the presence of metastases in lymph nodes.

Findings at EUS
Five studies have reported on the results of T and N staging of early-stage gastric adenocarcinoma [14,18–21].

T stage. From these studies, it can be concluded that the combined accuracy of T1 staging is 83% (Table 3.3). In more detail, the combined sensitivity of

Table 3.3 Reported endoscopic ultrasound (EUS) results on T staging in patients with early gastric cancer (GC).

Author	N	Biopsy result (n)	Probe (MHz)	Sensitivity T1 (%)	Specificity T1 (%)	Sensitivity T1m (%)	Specificity T1m (%)	Sensitivity T1sm (%)	Specificity T1sm (%)
Akahoshi et al. [18]	78	GC (78)	15	Acc.: 52/78 (67)		40/57 (70)		6/13 (46)	
Yanai et al. [14]	52	GC (52)	20	Acc.: 37/52 (71)		21/33 (64)		11/17 (65)	
Ohashi et al. [19]	49	GC (49)	7.5/12	Acc.: 39/49 (80)		37/38 (97)		2/11 (18)	
Yoshida et al. [20]	295	GC (295)	7.5/12/ 15/20/30	Acc.: 265/295 (90)		T1m+T1sm1: 246/264 (93)		T1sm2–3: 19/31 (61)	
Tsendsuren et al. [21]	12	GC (12)	5/7.5	Acc.: 10/12 (83)					
Total	486	GC (486)		Acc.: 403/486 (83)		98/128 (77)		19/41 (46)	

T1m gastric cancer was 77% (Table 3.3). One study reported the combined sensitivity of T1m *plus* T1sm1 (tumor invading the first of three layers of the submucosa) gastric cancers and found a sensitivity of 93% (246/264) for EUS [20]. The combined sensitivity of T1sm tumors was only 46%. The sensitivity of T1sm2–3 gastric cancers was somewhat higher, i.e. 61% (19/31) in this study [20]. These results suggest that the distinction between T1m and T1sm early gastric cancer is more difficult than when the cut-off point is set between the first and second layer of the submucosa. Nonetheless, even if invading only the first layer of the T1sm1, a distinction should be made between tumor invasion that is shallower or deeper than 400 µm. In the experience of these authors [20], well-differentiated gastric adenocarcinoma was not associated with lymph node metastases, provided that invasion was shallower than 400 µm into the submucosa.

Akahoshi *et al.* [18] investigated whether staging accuracy was influenced by endosocopic tumor type, histologic type, and tumor size. The accuracy in determining depth of invasion in relation to endoscopic type was significantly higher for the elevated type (91%) than for the depressed type of early cancer (56%). The staging accuracy classified by histologic type was significantly higher for differentiated (86%) than for undifferentiated (18%) cancer and decreased when tumor size increased.

As stated above, it is technically often difficult to make a distinction between mucosal and submucosal early gastric cancers. Matsumoto *et al.* [22] evaluated EUS images of the 3rd hyperechoic layer (submucosa) of 75 patients to define EUS features suggestive of submucosal tumor invasion. They found that irregular narrowing (60%), a budding sign (86%), meaning an irregularly bordered low echo break into the 3rd layer within a width of 2 mm below the tumor, or the combination of these features (91%) were predictive for the presence of submucosal invasion when tumorous changes in the 3rd layer exceeded 1 mm in depth.

These results show, as in early esophageal cancer, that EUS tends to overstage rather than to understage. In one study, the percentage of overstaging (false-positive ingrowth into the submucosa) was 43% [14], whereas in another study this was 24% for both early (*n*=12) and advanced (*n*=29) gastric cancer [21]. Similar to early esophageal cancer, this will result in a decision to perform a (subtotal) gastrectomy in these patients, which is in fact not desirable as an EMR would have been sufficient in the majority of these people.

N stage.   For N staging in early gastric cancer, EUS with high-frequency probes is inadequate, with one study reporting accuracy of 80%, but a sensitivity of 17% [18]. In the combined early and advanced gastric cancer series, sensitivity was still only 66% using a low-frequency EUS probe [21] (Table 3.4). Therefore, the presently available catheter probes are unreliable in detecting lymph node

Table 3.4 Reported endoscopic ultrasound (EUS) results on N staging in patients with early gastric cancer (GC).

Author	N	Biopsy result (*n*)	Probe (MHz)	Sensitivity N stage (%)	Specificity N stage (%)	PPV N stage	NPV N stage
Akahoshi *et al.* [18]	78	GC (78)	15	1/6 (17) (Acc.: 80%)	36/40 (90)	20%	88%
Tsendsuren *et al.* [21]	41	GC (41), both early (12) and advanced (29) cancer	5/7.5	27/41 (66)			

NPV: negative predictive value; PPV: positive predictive value.

metastases in early gastric cancer. The reason is that only perigastric lymph nodes near the lesion can be visualized, while deeper metastatic lymph nodes remain out of reach of these probes.

Conclusion

EUS using small caliber EUS probes can be used to try to discriminate between T1m and T1sm early gastric cancer. However, it is unreliable in detecting lymph nodes (N stage). Various tumor characteristics, for example a depressed tumor type as seen by endoscopy, an undifferentiated adenocarcinoma as seen by histology, and a larger tumor size negatively influence reliability of T staging. For the most optimal staging result, particularly of T stage, EUS should be combined with endoscopy to evaluate the macroscopic tumor type. Magnification endoscopy with dye spraying may play a role in the evaluation of the horizontal spread of the lesion. Endoscopic treatment of early gastric cancer should only be offered if the lesion is limited to the mucosa (T1m1–3) and in selected submucosal (T1sm1) tumors.

Colorectum

It has convincingly been shown that the early detection and endoscopic resection of precursor lesions in the colorectum is able to disrupt the adenoma-carcinoma sequence. Until recently, it was assumed that the majority of these precursor lesions were polypoid structures, which can easily be removed by snare polypectomy. However, as in Japan, flat and depressed non-polypoid colorectal lesions are increasingly being detected in Western patients and these accounted for 38% of all adenomas detected in a recent UK series [23]. Moreover, an anatomical preponderance of flat and depressed adenomas and carcinomas in the right colon has been demonstrated.

EMR is now increasingly being practised for flat and depressed lesions in the colorectum. These lesions are however associated with a higher submucosal invasion rate than polypoid lesions. Lymph nodes metastases have been reported in 15–50% of flat and depressed colorectal lesions invading the submucosal layers 2 + 3 (T1sm2–3). Lymph node metastases in intramucosal (T1m1–2) and focally extending submucosal (T1m3–sm1) cancer are rarely found and can therefore be treated by EMR [24].

Videoendoscopy

As the newer diagnostic endoscopic techniques are relatively time consuming and not generally available in many endoscopy units, it could be a more cost-effective and convenient approach if the discrimination between flat and depressed type T1m–sm1 and T1sm2–3 cancers could be made by videocolonoscopy.

Saitoh *et al.* [25] diagnosed and treated 64 depressed-type early CRCs using an Olympus GIF-2T200 endoscope or a Hitachi EVC-400-HM endoscope. When a faint abnormality of the mucosa was suspected by routine colonoscopy, 0.1% indigo carmine solution was sprayed onto the mucosal surface. Colonoscopic findings of T1m–sm1 cancers and more extended submucosal (sm2–3) cancers were compared with confirmed histologic findings. Characteristic colonoscopic findings for T1sm2–3 CRCs were: (1) an expansive appearance, (2) a deep depression surface, (3) an irregular bottom of depression surface, and (4) two or more mucosal folds converging toward the tumor. Using these findings, the invasion depth of depressed-type early CRC could be correctly determined in 58 of 64 lesions (91%).

Magnification endoscopy

Hurlstone *et al.* [26] used high magnification chromoscopic colonoscopy (HMCC) for discriminating neoplastic from non-neoplastic colorectal lesions, particularly when flat and depressed. Total colonoscopy was performed in 1850 patients using an Olympus C240Z magnifying colonoscope. The detailed non-magnified chromoscopic appearance of all lesions was documented using the macroscopic classification of the Japanese Research Society for Cancer of the Colon and Rectum, after delineating the contour with 0.5% indigo carmine [27]. The magnified surface pit pattern was then further classified according to Kudo's modified criteria (type I–V) [28]. A total of 1008 flat lesions were identified. Sensitivity and specificity of HMCC in distinguishing between non-neoplastic and neoplastic lesions were 98% and 92%, respectively. However, when using this technique to differentiate non-invasive from invasive neoplastic lesions, sensitivity was poor (50%) with a specificity of 98%. Therefore, HMCC is able to discriminate neoplastic from non-neoplastic lesions, but cannot be used to discriminate invasive from non-invasive neoplastic lesions.

Endoscopic ultrasound

Anatomy of the normal colonic wall
On EUS, the colonic wall is no different from the gastric wall in that it has a five-layered architecture. The 5th hyperechoic layer represents the serosa, including the subserosa, and in the rectum the adventitia. Using a high-resolution EUS probe, the fine hypoechoic layer (about 0.2 mm in thickness) between the 2nd and the 3rd hyperechoic layers in the colon also represents the muscularis mucosae separating the mucosa from the submucosa.

Findings at EUS

Eight studies have reported on the results of T and N staging of early stage colorectal carcinoma [29–36]. The majority of these lesions were flat or depressed early CRCs.

T stage.   Taking these studies together, we found that the combined accuracy of T1 staging is 90% (Table 3.5). Only one study reported on the sensitivity of T1m lesions and found this to be 88% [34]. Akasu *et al.* [30] performed the largest study (309 patients with HGD, or T1/T2 CRC) and made a distinction between T1sm1 and T1sm2–3 tumors. They found that the accuracy of a radial scanning transducer for the former was 96%, whereas this was 97% for tumors invading the deeper submucosa.

N stage.   For N staging in early CRC, EUS with high-frequency probes seems inadequate, with a reported accuracy varying between 24% and 89%, and a disappointingly low sensitivity of 9% [31] and 38% [30] in two studies, but a sensitivity of 80% in the most recent study by Hurlstone *et al.* [36] (Table 3.6). Given the rather superficial scanning capacity of these high-frequency EUS probes, it is not surprising that in the former two studies low sensitivity rates were found. On the other hand, specificity of EUS is high, suggesting that false-positive findings are unlikely.

EUS vs. high magnification chromoscopic colonoscopy

As a consequence of the findings summarized above, it is of particular interest to compare EUS with HMCC. Is one of these staging methods superior to the other or do they both have additional value in staging early CRC?

Both Matsumoto *et al.* [31] and Hurlstone *et al.* [36] compared HMCC with high-frequency 20/12 MHz miniprobe EUS. In both studies, it was found that the accuracy for invasive submucosal depth (T1sm2–3) detection was significantly higher with EUS than with HMCC, i.e. 92% vs. 63% [31] and 93% vs. 59% [36], respectively. Negative predictive value for deep invasion was also higher for EUS than for HMCC (91% vs. 54% [31] and 88% and 47% [36], respectively). The accuracy for lymph node metastasis was however surprisingly different between the two studies, 24% for EUS and 72% for HMCC in the study by Matsumoto *et al.* [31] vs. 85% for EUS and 44% for HMCC in the study by Hurlstone *et al.* [36]. This is remarkable, but the impressive results for lymph node detection by Hurlstone *et al.* [36] have not been reported previously and have not been confirmed by others so far (Table 3.6). These two studies provide evidence that high-frequency probe EUS imaging is a more sensitive and more specific tool for establishing invasive depth in T1sm CRC. The results in the study of Matsumoto *et al.* [31] suggest that HMCC may be predictive for lymph nodes metastasis in early-stage CRC, but further trials are required.

Table 3.5 Reported endoscopic ultrasound (EUS) results on T staging in patients with early colorectal cancer (CRC).

Author	N	Biopsy result (n)	Probe (MHz)	Sensitivity T1 (%)	Specificity T1 (%)	Sensitivity T1m (%)	Specificity T1m (%)	Sensitivity T1sm1 (%)	Specificity T1sm1 (%)	Sensitivity T1sm2–3 (%)	Specificity T1sm2–3 (%)
Saitoh et al. [29]	49	Flat/depressed CRC (49)	20	Acc.: 43/49 (88)							
Akasu et al. [30]	309	Rectal cancer (Tis-T2) (309)	7.5/12					270/274 (99) (Acc.: 96%)	26/35 (74)	261/266 (98) (Acc.: 97%)	38/43 (88)
Matsumoto et al. [31]	50	Flat/depressed CRC (50)	12/20	Acc.: 45/49 (92)						25/28 (89)	20/22 (91)
Tseng et al. [32]	10	CRC (T1) (10)	12 (+balloon)	Acc.: 10/10 (100)							
Stergiou et al. [33]	33	Adenoma (16) CRC (T1) (17)	12	Acc.: 33/33 (100)							
Konishi et al. [34]	125	Villous (35)	7.5	Villous: Acc.: 21/35 (60)		Villous: 18/20 (60)		Villous: ½ (50)			
		Non-villous (90) (T1/T2)		Non-villous: Acc.: 82/90 (91)		Non-villous: 18/21 (86)		Non-villous: 8/11 (73)			
Hurlstone et al. [35]	48	Flat/depressed (Tis/T1) (48)	12.5	Acc.: 48/48 (100)							
Hurlstone et al. [36]	52	Flat/depressed (T1sm1–3) (52)	12.5/20	Acc.: 49/52 (94)							
Total	676			Acc.: 331/366 (90)		36/41 (88)		279/287 (97)	26/35 (74)	286/294 (97)	58/67 (87)

Table 3.6 Reported endoscopic ultrasound (EUS) results on N staging in patients with early colorectal cancer (CRC).

Author	N	Biopsy result (n)	Probe (MHz)	Sensitivity N stage (%)	Specificity N stage (%)	PPV N stage (%)	NPV N stage (%)
Akasu et al. [30]	309	Rectal cancer (Tis-T1) (309)	7.5/12	3/8 (38) (Acc.: 89%)	68/72 (94)	3/8 (38)	68/73 (93)
Matsumoto et al. [31]	50	Flat/depressed CRC (50)	12/20	2/23 (9) (Acc.: 24%)	5/6 (83)		
Hurlstone et al. [36]	52	Flat/depressed (T1sm1–3) (52)	12.5/20	8/10 (80) (Acc.: 85%)	15/17 (88)	8/10 (80)	15/17 (88)
Total	411			13/41 (32)	88/95 (93)		

NPV: negative predictive value; PPV: positive predictive value.

Conclusion

EUS is the preferred method of discriminating between flat and depressed T1m/T1sm1 CRC and T1sm2–3 CRC, however EUS is less reliable in detecting lymph nodes. HMCC can be used to discriminate neoplastic from non-neoplastic lesions. Both procedures provide complementary information with respect to the decision to perform a local or a surgical treatment. It remains to be established whether videoendoscopy *plus* chromoendoscopy if an abnormality of the mucosa is suspected can replace high magnification endoscopy. For this, additional trials are indicated.

Conclusion

Staging of early-stage neoplastic lesions in the GI tract is a part of the work-up of patients with these disorders as it is able to direct a treatment decision toward a local endoscopic treatment with EMR or more radical surgical therapy. In general, EUS with high-frequency EUS probes is the preferred technique to accurately stage early malignancies in the esophagus, stomach, and colorectum. The role of HRE and high magnification endoscopy lies primarily in detecting these lesions. Both modalities play only a modest role in staging early neoplastic lesions in the GI tract. Finally, EMR is a safe procedure and can, apart from being a therapeutic procedure, also be used as a diagnostic procedure making the staging of early lesions in some cases unnecessary.

References

1 May A, Gunter E, Roth F *et al.* Accuracy of staging in early oesophageal cancer using high resolution endoscopy and high resolution endosonography: a comparative, prospective, and blinded trial. *Gut* 2004; **53**: 634–40.
2 Araki K, Ohno S, Egashira A *et al.* Pathologic features of superficial esophageal squamous cell carcinoma with lymph node and distal metastasis. *Cancer* 2002; **94**: 570–5.
3 Westerterp M, Koppert LB, Buskens CJ *et al.* Outcome of surgical treatment for early adenocarcinoma of the esophagus or gastro-esophageal junction. *Virchows Arch* 2005; **446**: 497–504.
4 Rice TW, Blackstone EH, Goldblum JR *et al.* Superficial adenocarcinoma of the esophagus. *J Thorac Cardiovasc Surg* 2001; **122**: 1077–90.
5 Catalano MF, Sivak MV Jr, Rice T *et al.* Endosonographic features predictive of lymph node metastasis. *Gastrointest Endosc* 1994; **40**: 442–6.
6 Vazquez-Sequeiros E. Nodal staging: number or site of nodes? How to improve accuracy? Is FNA always necessary? Junctional tumors – what's N and what's M? *Endoscopy* 2006; **38** Suppl 1: S4–8.
7 Scotiniotis IA, Kochman ML, Lewis JD *et al.* Accuracy of EUS in the evaluation of Barrett's esophagus and high-grade dysplasia or intramucosal carcinoma. *Gastrointest Endosc* 2001; **54**: 689–96.
8 Buskens CJ, Westerterp M, Lagarde SM *et al.* Prediction of appropriateness of local endoscopic treatment for high-grade dysplasia and early adenocarcinoma by EUS and histopathologic features. *Gastrointest Endosc* 2004; **60**: 703–10.
9 Larghi A, Lightdale CJ, Memeo L *et al.* EUS followed by EMR for staging of high-grade dysplasia and early cancer in Barrett's esophagus. *Gastrointest Endosc* 2005; **62**: 16–23.

10 Waxman I, Raju GS, Critchlow J et al. High-frequency probe ultrasonography has limited accuracy for detecting invasive adenocarcinoma in patients with Barrett's esophagus and high-grade dysplasia or intramucosal carcinoma: a case series. *Am J Gastroenterol* 2006; **101:** 1773–9.

11 Pech O, May A, Gunter E et al. The impact of endoscopic ultrasound and computed tomography on the TNM staging of early cancer in Barrett's esophagus. *Am J Gastroenterol* 2006; **101:** 2223–9.

12 Shimoyama S, Imamura K, Takeshita Y et al. The useful combination of a higher frequency miniprobe and endoscopic submucosal dissection for the treatment of T1 esophageal cancer. *Surg Endosc* 2006; **20:** 434–8.

13 Kelly S, Harris KM, Berry E et al. A systematic review of the staging performance of endoscopic ultrasound in gastro-oesophageal carcinoma. *Gut* 2001; **49:** 534–9.

14 Yanai H, Noguchi T, Mizumacchi S et al. A blind comparison of the effectiveness of endoscopic ultrasonography and endoscopy in staging early gastric cancer. *Gut* 1999; **44:** 361–5.

15 Guelrud M, Herrera I, Essenfeld H et al. Enhanced magnification endoscopy: a new technique to identify specialized intestinal metaplasia in Barrett's esophagus. *Gastrointest Endosc* 2001; **53:** 559–65.

16 Tanaka K, Toyoda H, Kadowaki S et al. Features of early gastric cancer and gastric adenoma by enhanced-magnification endoscopy. *J Gastroenterol* 2006; **41:** 332–8.

17 Sano T, Kobori O, Muto T. Lymph node metastasis from early gastric cancer: endoscopic resection of tumour. *Br J Surg* 1992; **79:** 241–4.

18 Akahoshi K, Chijiiwa Y, Hamada S et al. Pretreatment staging of endoscopically early gastric cancer with a 15MHz ultrasound catheter probe. *Gastrointest Endosc* 1998; **48:** 470–6.

19 Ohashi S, Segawa K, Okamura S et al. The utility of endoscopic ultrasonography and endoscopy in the endoscopic mucosal resection of early gastric cancer. *Gut* 1999; **45:** 599–604.

20 Yoshida S, Tanaka S, Kunihiro K et al. Diagnostic ability of high-frequency ultrasound probe sonography in staging early gastric cancer, especially for submucosal invasion. *Abdom Imaging* 2005; **30:** 518–23.

21 Tsendsuren T, Jun SM, Mian XH. Usefulness of endoscopic ultrasonography in preoperative TNM staging of gastric cancer. *World J Gastroenterol* 2006; **12:** 43–7.

22 Matsumoto Y, Yanai H, Tokiyama H, et al. Endosonographic ultrasonography for diagnosis of submucosal invasion in early gastric cancer. *J Gastroenterol* 2000; **35:** 326–31.

23 Hurlstone DP, Cross SS, Adam I et al. A prospective clinicopathological and endoscopic evaluation of flat and depressed colorectal lesions in the United Kingdom. *Am J Gastroenterol* 2003; **98:** 2543–9.

24 Kurahashi T, Kaneko K, Makino R et al. Colorectal carcinoma with special reference to growth pattern classifications: clinicopathologic characteristics and genetic changes. *J Gastroenterol* 2002; **37:** 354–62.

25 Saitoh Y, Obara T, Watari J et al. Invasion depth diagnosis of depressed type early colorectal cancers by combined use of videoendoscopy and chromoendoscopy. *Gastrointest Endosc* 1998; **48:** 362–70.

26 Hurlstone DP, Sanders DS, Cross SS et al. Colonoscopic resection of lateral spreading tumours: a prospective analysis of endoscopic mucosal resection. *Gut* 2004; **53:** 1334–9.

27 Japanese Research Society for Cancer of the Colon and Rectum. General rules for clinical and pathological studies on cancer of the colon, rectum and anus. Part I. Clinical classification. *Jpn J Surg* 1983; **13:** 557–73.

28 Kudo S, Rubio CA, Teixeira CR et al. Pit pattern in colorectal neoplasia: endoscopic magnifying view. *Endoscopy* 2001; **33:** 367–73.

29 Saitoh Y, Obara T, Einami K et al. Efficacy of high-frequency ultrasound probes for the preoperative staging of invasion depth in flat and depressed colorectal tumors. *Gastrointest Endosc* 1996; **44:** 34–9.

30 Akasu T, Kondo H, Moriya Y et al. Endorectal ultrasonography and treatment of early stage rectal cancer. *World J Surg* 2000; **24:** 1061–8.

31 Matsumoto T, Hizawa K, Esaki M et al. Comparison of EUS and magnifying colonoscopy for assessment of small colorectal cancers. *Gastrointest Endosc* 2002; **56:** 354–60.

32 Tseng LJ, Jao YT, Mo LR. Preoperative staging of colorectal cancer with a balloon-sheathed miniprobe. *Endoscopy* 2002; **34**: 564–8.

33 Stergiou N, Haji-Kermani N, Schneider C *et al.* Staging of colonic neoplasms by colonoscopic miniprobe ultrasonography. *Int J Colorectal Dis* 2003; **18**: 445–9.

34 Konishi K, Akita Y, Kaneko K *et al.* Evaluation of endoscopic ultrasonography in colorectal villous lesions. *Int J Colorectal Dis* 2003; **18**: 19–24.

35 Hurlstone DP, Brown S, Cross SS *et al.* Endoscopic ultrasound miniprobe staging of colorectal cancer: can management be modified? *Endoscopy* 2005; **37**: 710–14.

36 Hurlstone DP, Brown S, Cross SS *et al.* High magnification chromoscopic colonoscopy or high frequency 20 MHz mini probe endoscopic ultrasound staging for early colorectal neoplasia: a comparative prospective analysis. *Gut* 2005; **54**: 1585–9.

CHAPTER 4

Advances in Endoscopic Imaging of Barrett's Esophagus

AMITABH CHAK AND FAREES T. FAROOQ

Introduction

Barrett's esophagus (BE) is defined by displacement of the squamocolumnar junction proximal to the esophagogastric junction *and* the presence of metaplastic intestinal-type epithelium in place of the normal esophageal squamous epithelium. As this definition suggests, the diagnosis of BE requires both endoscopic findings and histologic confirmation. It seems intuitive that techniques aimed to improve endoscopic detection or aid in histologic prediction would be beneficial.

The importance of BE is clearly based on the recognition of it as a precursor of esophageal adenocarcinoma. The histologic progression from metaplastic BE to dysplastic BE and subsequently to adenocarcinoma is the rationale for endoscopic screening and surveillance programs. Current surveillance protocols call for periodic endoscopic examination for mucosal abnormalities as well as four-quadrant random biopsies every 1–2 cm within a segment of BE. The limitations of such protocols include sampling error because they sample less than 1% of the affected esophageal surface as well as the monotony and time required to perform biopsies in this fashion. The development of endoscopic imaging modalities that identify intestinal metaplasia and facilitate differentiation of bland Barrett's epithelium from low-grade and high-grade dysplasia and early adenocarcinoma has been the focus of intense research. The potential merit of such imaging modalities is the possibility of complete examination of a BE segment for dysplasia without the need for biopsy or with the ability to focus biopsies to areas most likely to contain dysplastic epithelium. A number of endoscopic imaging methods have been developed for this purpose over the past two decades. The basis for each method, as well as the

Endoscopic Mucosal Resection. Edited by M. Conio, P. Siersema, A. Repici and T. Ponchon. © 2008 Blackwell Publishing. ISBN 978-1-4051-5885-5.

technique, interpretation, and evidence for these imaging modalities, is the focus of this chapter.

Histopathology in Barrett's esophagus

To understand how these novel imaging methods might enhance the ability to identify intestinal metaplasia and dysplasia and to realize their limitations it is necessary to understand the histologic criteria that define Barrett's esophagus and its dysplastic stages. Normally, the esophagus has a stratified squamous epithelium with a uniformly flat surface. The hallmark of Barrett's esophagus is specialized intestinal metaplasia, which contains absorptive goblet cells arranged in a villous architecture. Thus, imaging techniques can identify Barrett's epithelium either by its absorptive nature or by magnifying to a resolution that identifies its villous structure. Low-grade dysplasia is characterized by increased nuclear activity that results in variations in nuclear size, nuclear crowding, and some loss of epithelial polarity. In vivo recognition of low-grade dysplasia requires an image resolution that identifies nuclei or a chemical method that identifies increased nuclear activity. In high-grade dysplasia (HGD) and early cancer, not only is there increased nuclear activity, but the villous architecture is distorted. Therefore, imaging techniques that can identify epithelial architecture are able to resolve these changes.

Overview of endoscopic imaging for Barrett's esophagus

One of the difficulties in identifying dyplastic foci in BE is the large esophageal surface area that must be examined. In general, imaging methods with higher resolution that provide greater tissue detail or histologic information are difficult, if not impossible, to apply in scanning an entire segment of BE. Lower resolution methods can usually be used to image the entire esophagus but are less reliable in distinguishing dysplastic from non-dysplastic epithelium. The ideal imaging technique would have the following characteristics: high sensitivity for dysplasia, moderate specificity not affected by inflammation, the ability to scan a wide area in real time, high inter-observer agreement, ability to localize dysplastic areas for biopsy, and non-prohibitive cost. No single currently available imaging method has all of these criteria or even several of these criteria. However, the development of new endoscopic imaging techniques has opened exciting avenues in the area of Barrett's research with the potential to improve upon surveillance and treatment strategies that comprise the current standard of care. In the future, we may find that the combination of various imaging methods is the best management algorithm.

Endoscopic imaging methods

Chromoendoscopy

Chromoendoscopy refers to the application of contrast stains to the mucosa at endoscopy such that surface patterns are highlighted. The use of various contrast agents including methylene blue, acetic acid, Lugol's solution, and indigo carmine has been described extensively in the literature.

Methylene blue (MB) is absorbed by intestinal-type epithelium. Therefore, application of methylene blue in the setting of BE results in staining of Barrett's epithelium with sparing of non-intestinal columnar and squamous epithelium. Furthermore, dysplastic Barrett's epithelium stains less than BE without dysplasia due to the paucity of goblet cells in the setting of dysplasia. Therefore, areas of BE with dysplasia may be more evident on chromoendoscopy using MB. The technique of chromoendoscopy using MB involves clearance of surface mucus in the esophagus by flushing with 10% N-acetylcysteine. Subsequently, 0.5% MB is applied to the esophageal mucosa using an endoscopic spray catheter. After a 2-minute staining period, excess MB is cleared by flushing with sterile water. The use of MB has been described extensively in the literature. The results of these studies have been quite variable. Some authors have reported favorable results, some have reported mixed results, and some have reported unfavorable results [1–3]. This variability may be related to the fact that this technique is quite observer dependent and also may reflect some publication bias in the earlier reports.

The methylene blue chromoendoscopy technique has not been adopted widely and recent studies have suggested that methylene blue chromoendoscopy is likely to be of limited benefit in BE surveillance.

Unlike methylene blue, indigo carmine is simply a contrast agent that accentuates mucosal surface patterns. Indigo carmine is applied during endoscopy using a typical endoscopic spray catheter, after clearing of surface mucus with a water, saline, or N-acetylcysteine flush. The use of a cap fitted at the endoscope tip has been described to stabilize high magnification images and image areas of interest. Sharma *et al.* [4] have investigated the surface patterns in Barrett's esophagus using magnification chromoendoscopy with Indigo carmine. In their study of 80 patients with BE, three distinct surface patterns were appreciated: ridged/villous, circular, and irregular/distorted. The ridged/villous pattern, which has a cerebriform appearance, and the circular pattern, which has uniform circular or oval areas were observed in non-dysplastic BE and in low-grade dysplasia. The irregular/distorted pattern was observed in HGD with a 100% sensitivity and specificity.

Narrow-band imaging

Conventional videoendoscopes transmit white light from a xenon lamp that passes through a rotating red-green-blue filter. The transmitted light, composed of alternating pulses of red, green, and blue light, illuminates the imaged area, and the wavelengths of visible light waves that strike and are absorbed or reflected by the imaged area are detected by a charge-coupled device (CCD) at the endoscope tip. The light waves detected by the CCD are transmitted to the video processor unit where superimposed red, green, and blue light images are integrated to create the final videoendoscopic image that is detected by the human eye [5]. In narrow-band imaging (NBI), an additional special filter has been incorporated into the endoscope such that imaged tissue is illuminated with narrow band-pass ranges of light in the red, green, and blue spectra. Blue light is disproportionately transmitted whereas other light wavelengths are selectively removed by absorption and/or interference. Red light at a wavelength of 650 nm penetrates tissue more deeply than blue light of 475 nm wavelength. Therefore, blue light is theoretically better for imaging superficial tissue structures in detail than red light or white light which is comprised of the entire visible light spectrum. As a result, the use of NBI allows for higher resolution of superficial tissue structures. In addition, blue light is preferentially absorbed by hemoglobin. Therefore, hemoglobin-containing structures, such as capillaries and luminal blood, are accentuated in the presence of blue light [6–9].

The value of NBI in the evaluation of gastrointestinal mucosal lesions, including colonic polyps and Barrett's esophagus, has been investigated. Sharma *et al.* studied the mucosal and vascular patterns in Barrett's esophagus [8,9]. The study found three distinct mucosal patterns in patients with BE. The ridge/villous pattern, as also identified in their high-magnification chromoendoscopy studies, is characterized by uniformly aligned ridges alternating with a villiform pattern. The ridge/villous pattern is seen as alternating dark and light lines on NBI. The circular pattern is characterized by a uniformly arranged circular mucosal pattern. The irregular/distorted pattern demonstrated ridge and villous pattern irregularity and distortion. Vascular patterns on NBI were characterized as normal (thin, uniformly branching vessels) or abnormal (dilated, corkscrew vessels in non-uniform branching patterns). Using a magnification NBI endoscope fitted with a cap to stabilize a focused imaged area, Sharma *et al.* found a positive predictive value, sensitivity, and specificity of 93.5%, 86.5%, and 94.7% for the ridge/villous pattern in BE without HGD and 100%, 98.7%, and 95.3% for the irregular/distorted pattern in BE with HGD [9]. The positive predictive value, sensitivity, and specificity of the abnormal vascular pattern for HGD was 94.7%, 100%, and 97.4%. The false-positives with an abnormal vascular pattern included two areas of low-grade dysplasia. Normal vascular patterns were found in areas of nondysplastic BE, low-grade dysplasia, and intestinal metaplasia of the gastric cardia. Kara *et al.* [6] also characterized BE based on mucosal and vascular patterns. Their terminology was slightly different from that used by Sharma *et al.* but essentially described the same findings. In this study, irregular or disrupted mucosal pattern, irregular vascular pattern, and the presence of abnormal blood vessels were independent predictors of HGD ($p < 0.05$). This study also found a new pattern, a flat featureless epithelium with long normal capillaries that also corresponded to non-dysplastic BE.

Autofluorescence

Fluorescence is the process in which certain molecules, termed fluorophores, absorb light energy and reach an excited state. From the excited state, fluorophores return to the ground state and, in that process, emit light of a longer wavelength than the light that produced the excited state. Emitted light within the visible light spectrum accounts for the optical phenomenon of fluorescence. The use of fluorescence for imaging may be based on endogenous fluorophores such as nicotinamide adenine dinucleotide (NADH) or collagen or the use of exogenously supplied fluorophores, such as porfimer sodium or the fluorescent dye fluorescein. The exploitation of endogenous fluorophores in biological tissue for imaging is termed autofluorescence [10]. Variations in molecular composition

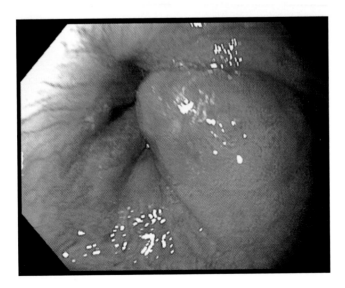

Fig. 4.1 Barrett's esophagus with high-grade dysplasia on standard white-light videoendoscopy.

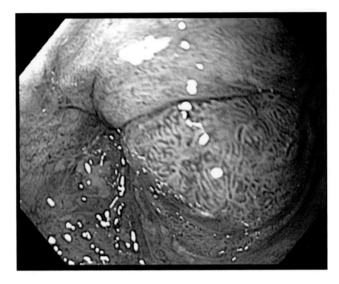

Fig. 4.2 The same area with NBI. An irregular/distorted mucosal pattern is apparent in an area of high-grade dysplasia.

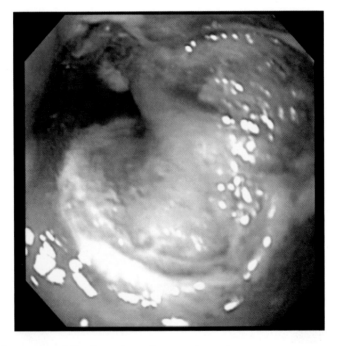

Fig. 4.3 The same area following endoscopic mucosal resection.

and tissue microstructure lead to differences in fluorescence, thereby creating the potential for distinguishing neoplastic from non-neoplastic tissue. Prototype endoscopes that make use of this technology have been developed in recent years. Additional tissue characteristics based on red and green light reflectance have also been incorporated to improve the image production algorithm. The application of the concept of autofluorescence using the endoscope as the source of excitation light waves has been termed light-induced fluorescence endoscopy (LIFE).

Early fiberoptic endoscopy technology that incorporated LIFE found that inflammation as well as dysplasia leads to increased autofluorescence. The autofluorescence signal is also quite weak and difficult to identify, limiting the applicability of this technology for BE surveillance. The use of intravenous or topical fluorophores such as 5-aminolevulinic acid improved the performance of LIFE but still not to a level where it could be applied clinically [11]. Kara et al. [12] compared autofluorescence-targeted biopsies with random four-quadrant biopsies in 50 patients presenting for BE surveillance. Using a fiber-optic endoscope with the LIFE II autofluorescence system (Xillix Corp, British Columbia, Canada), the investigators found that the use of LIFE-targeted biopsies did not improve the detection of HGD and adenocarcinoma over standard white-light endoscopy with the 'Seattle protocol'.

The value of autofluorescence endoscopy in the detection of dysplasia in Barrett's esophagus has been improved by the development of new AFI techniques that utilize CCD endoscopes and imaging algorithms that incorporate reflectance. In another study, investigators from Amsterdam used a prototype autofluorescence imaging (AFI) system (Olympus, Inc., Tokyo, Japan) that integrates autofluorescence and red/green reflectance to produce a real-time AFI image in which non-dysplastic Barrett's esophagus appears green and suspected dysplastic Barrett's esophagus appears blue/violet [13]. In this initial unblinded pilot study, the investigators compared the rate of detection of HGD in all-comers being evaluated with BE using AFI-guided biopsies and random four-quadrant biopsies. In 60 patients, AFI-guided biopsies increased the detection rate of HGD or adenocarcinoma from 23% to 33%. The positive predictive value of AFI-suspicious areas was 49% while the negative predictive value was 89%.

The same investigators later studied 20 patients with known BE with HGD and identified suspicious areas using AFI and NBI [14]. Biopsies obtained from these areas were used to determine the accuracy of histologic prediction based on AFI. They found that the false-positive rate of AFI for predicting dysplasia was 40%. Additional interpretation of NBI along the AFI reduced false-positivity to 10%.

Thus, similar to NBI, autoflourescence endoscopy is conceptually interesting and shows promise as an adjunctive imaging method. However, the early data show that AFI lacks the sensitivity and specificity to warrant routine use in

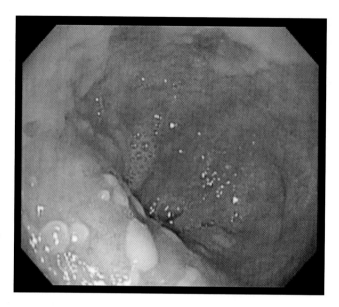

Fig. 4.4   Barrett's esophagus with standard white-light videoendoscopy.

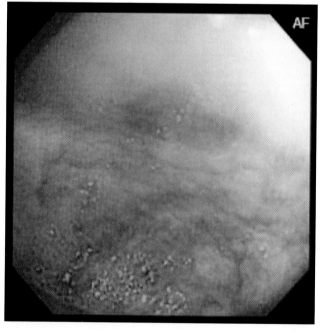

Fig. 4.5   The same area with autofluorescence imaging. Non-dyplastic BE appears green, while high-grade dysplasia appears violet.

guiding endoscopic surveillance [15]. As AFI instruments continue to evolve, these parameters are likely to improve. And, as Kara *et al.*'s studies suggest, the combination of imaging techniques such as AFI and NBI may ultimately be the most accurate way of detecting dysplastic BE.

Optical coherence tomography

Optical coherence tomography (OCT) is an imaging technique that is conceptually analogous to B-mode ultrasound, except that OCT uses light waves rather than sound waves. Light waves derived from a low-coherence light source are delivered to an optical-fiber splitter that sends half of the light to the area to be imaged and the other half to a reference mirror. By a process termed interferometry, the backscattered light from tissue and the time delay between reflected light waves from tissue and the reference mirror are processed [16–18]. The resulting image is a two-dimensional tomogram with a resolution of 1–15 μm and a scanning depth of 1–3 mm. OCT uses optical fiber technology allowing for incorporation into a catheter-probe design that can be passed through an endoscope channel. Although the resolution of OCT is not quite at the level of histopathology, the aim of OCT imaging, in contrast to chromoendoscopy, NBI, and AFI, is to produce images that provide some degree of histologic detail. In this context, OCT can not only differentiate Barrett's epithelium from squamous epithelium and detect villous/crypt architecture, but it also has the potential to differentiate non-dysplastic BE from dysplastic BE.

Studies in the colon polyp model were initially used to determine the OCT characteristics of dysplasia – loss of tissue organization and reduced light scattering, that have since been applied to the esophagus [19]. Using these criteria in a double-blinded, prospective study of 33 patients with BE, Isenberg *et al.* [20] found that in detecting dysplasia in BE, OCT had a sensitivity and specificity of 68% and 82%, respectively. Another study by Evans *et al.* [18] using analogous criteria found that OCT could be used to distinguish BE from non-metaplastic epithelium at the squamocolumnar junction. Currently available endoscopic OCT probes do not yet have the capability of providing images at the nuclear level and are applicable only for research purposes at this time. However, ongoing development of these devices with improved resolution is likely to improve the diagnostic accuracy of OCT in Barrett's esophagus.

Confocal endomicroscopy

As discussed earlier, fluorescence imaging is based on the emitted light from molecules returning from the excited state to ground state. In fluorescence

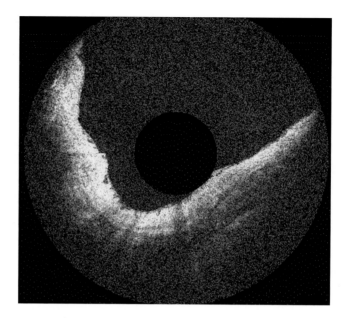

Fig. 4.6 OCT image of Barrett's esophagus. Villous surface pattern is apparent.

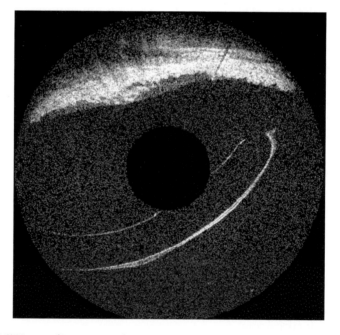

Fig. 4.7 OCT image of Barrett's esophagus with high-grade dysplasia characterized by loss of tissue organization. (The thin bright line near the center of the field represents the cap fitted at the endoscope tip.)

imaging an entire area is flooded with light, and a wide area of emitted light is detected. Fluorescence emitted by tissue away from the region of interest interferes with the resolution of the in-focus region. In confocal microscopy, laser light is reflected off a dichromatic mirror to an in-focus tissue plane. Exogenously supplied fluorophores within the imaged specimen emit light, and emitted light of sufficient wavelength is refocused through a pinhole at a conjugate plane to the imaged area. The pinhole aperture at the detector allows out-of-focus emitted light to be rejected whereas light transmitted though the pinhole is detected and processed to produce an 'optical section' of one focal plane within the imaged region of interest [21–23]. Scanning over multiple points allows construction of a two-dimensional planar image. The confocal microscope has been miniaturized such that it can be incorporated into the tip of an endoscope.

Confocal endomicroscopic images are of high resolution and allow for subsurface mucosal analysis and in vivo histology. Kiesslich *et al.* [24] imaged 63 patients with BE following administration of fluorescein. By confocal imaging, intestinal metaplasia was easily demonstrated by the presence of dark goblet cells, and low-grade neoplasia was identifiable by the presence of dark irregularly shaped epithelial cells. In addition subepithelial capillaries were detectable and differed in pattern between non-dysplastic BE and low-grade neoplasia. The accuracy of confocal endomicroscopy in detecting BE and low-grade neoplasia was 96.8% and 97.4%, respectively. Low-grade and high-grade dysplasia and early cancer were not specifically distinguished in this study. Therefore, the ability to distinguish non-dyplastic BE from BE with varying degrees of dysplasia short of early cancer is uncertain.

Endoscopic ultrasound (EUS)

While certainly not a new imaging method, EUS is worthy of mention in the context of BE imaging and endoscopic mucosal resection. EUS is used commonly for the staging of esophageal cancer, but the use of EUS for detection of early cancer in patients with dysplastic BE has not been universally accepted.

EUS in Barrett's esophagus can be performed using a standard radial-scanning echoendoscope or alternatively using high-frequency catheter probes. Neither method has been shown to be reliable in differentiating BE from BE with dysplasia, as the mucosal thickening seen in dysplasia is mimicked by inflammation in the setting of non-dysplastic BE. Furthermore, the compressability of the esophageal wall layers by the echoendoscope balloon increases the subjectivity of EUS interpretation for this indication. However, EUS may have a role in selecting patients with high-grade dysplasia or early cancer for endoscopic ablative therapy by determining the presence or absence of submucosal invasion and lymph node involvement [25–28].

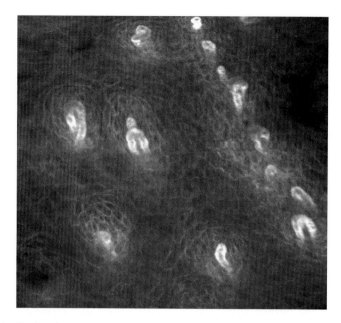

Fig. 4.8 Confocal endomicroscopic image of squamous epithelium in a patient with chronic gastroesophageal reflux disease showing normal squamous cells outlined faintly by fluorescein and fluorescein in the multiple interpapillary capillary loops. Red blood cells can be seen 'stacked' in the blood vessels.

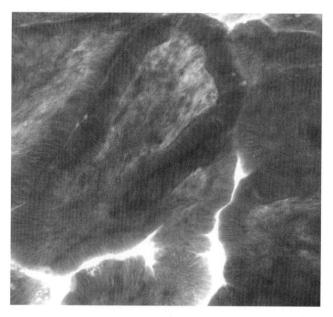

Fig. 4. 9 Confocal endomicroscopic image of Barrett's esophagus in the same patient as Fig. 4.8, showing the villiform intestinal-type epithelium with dark goblet cells after injection of intravenous fluorescein. Note the normal architecture of the glands, abundant lamina propria, intact basement membrane, and orderly arrangement of epithelial cells consistent with absence of dysplasia.

In a study of 25 patients referred for endoscopic therapy of BE with HGD or early cancer, EUS identified submucosal invasion or lymphadenopathy in 20% of patients, thereby altering their management from endoscopic therapy to surgery [27]. The use of EUS and CT staging for 100 patients referred for endoscopic therapy of BE with early cancer identified 23% of the patients as more appropriate for surgery than endoscopic ablation based on tumoral and nodal staging, with EUS far exceeding the sensitivity of CT in detecting advanced disease [26]. The results of these studies suggest that EUS staging should be strongly considered prior to undertaking EMR in a patient who is otherwise a good surgical candidate.

Conclusions

Identification of the ideal endoscopic method for surveillance of Barrett's esophagus and detection of dysplasia remains an elusive goal. Whether recent advances in endoscopic imaging such as NBI, OCT, and AFI will complement or replace some of the older methods of mucosal enhancement such as chromoendoscopy from a clinically practical standpoint is uncertain. What is clear is that the more sophisticated techniques such as OCT and confocal endomicroscopy which produce higher resolution images inevitably narrow the endoscopic 'field of view' making these techniques difficult to use in scanning an entire segment of BE. In the future, combining techniques that can image a large region and then focus in on suspicious areas for targeted biopsies or therapy (e.g. EMR) may be the optimal approach.

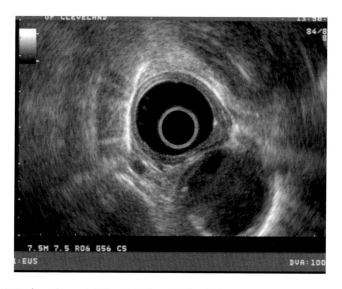

Fig. 4.10   EUS of esophagus in BE with high-grade dysplasia.

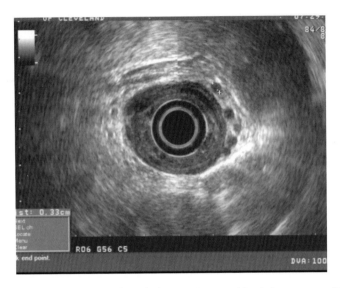

Fig. 4.11   EUS of esophagus in esophageal adenocarcinoma arising in long-segment Barrett's esophagus. Hypoechoic periesophageal lymph nodes are present.

Acknowledgments

The confocal endomicroscopy images were kindly provided by Marcia Canto, MD. The autofluorescence images were provided courtesy of Michelle Wong Kee Song, MD.

References

1 Lim CH, Rotimi O, Dexter SP, Axon AT. Randomized crossover study that used methylene blue or random 4-quadrant biopsy for the diagnosis of dysplasia in Barrett's esophagus. *Gastrointest Endosc* 2006; **64**: 195–9.
2 Egger K, Werner M, Meining A *et al.* Biopsy surveillance is still necessary in patients with Barrett's esophagus despite new endoscopic imaging techniques. *Gut* 2003; **52**: 18–23.
3 Canto MI, Kalloo A. Chromoendoscopy for Barrett's esophagus in the twenty-first century: to stain or not to stain? *Gastrointest Endosc* 2006; **64**: 200–4.
4 Sharma P, Weston AP, Topalovski M *et al.* Magnification chromoendoscopy for the detection of intestinal metaplasia and dysplasia in Barrett's oesophagus. *Gut* 2003; **52**: 24–7.
5 Kawahara I, Ichikawa H. Flexible endoscope technology. In: MV Sivak, ed. *Gastroenterologic Endoscopy*. WB Saunders, Philadelphia, PA, 2000: 16–29.
6 Kara MA, Ennahachi M, Fockens P. Detection and classification of the mucosal and vascular patterns (mucosal morphology) in Barrett's esophagus by using narrow band imaging. *Gastrointest Endosc* 2006; **64**: 155–66.
7 Hamamoto Y, Endo T, Nosho K *et al.* Usefulness of narrow-band imaging endoscopy for diagnosis of Barrett's esophagus. *J Gastroenterol* 2004; **39**: 14–20.
8 Sharma P, Bansal A, Mathur S *et al.* The utility of a novel narrow band imaging endoscopy system in patients with Barrett's esophagus. *Gastrointest Endosc* 2006; **64**: 167–75.
9 Sharma P, Marcon N, Wani S *et al.* Non-biopsy detection of intestinal metaplasia and dysplasia in Barrett's esophagus: a prospective multicenter study. *Endoscopy* 2006; **38**: 1206–12.

10 Kara MA, Bergman JJ. Autofluorescence imaging and narrow-band imaging for the detection of early neoplasia in patients with Barrett's esophagus. *Endoscopy* 2006; **38**: 627–31.

11 Messmann H, Knuchel R, Baumler W, Holstege A, Scholmerich J. Endoscopic fluorescence detection of dysplasia in patients with Barrett's esophagus, ulcerative colitis, or adenomatous polyps after 5-aminolevulinic acid-induced protoporphyrin IX sensitization. *Gastrointest Endosc* 1999; **49**: 97–101.

12 Kara MA, Smits ME, Rosmolen WD *et al*. A randomized crossover study comparing light-induced fluorescence endoscopy with standard videoendoscopy for the detection of early neoplasia in Barrett's esophagus. *Gastrointest Endosc* 2005; **61**: 671–8.

13 Kara MA, Peters FP, ten Kate FJ *et al*. Endoscopic video autofluorescence imaging may improve the detection of early neoplasia in patients with Barrett's esophagus. *Gastrointest Endosc* 2005; **61**: 679–85.

14 Kara MA, Peters FP, Fockens P *et al*. Endoscopic video-autofluoroescence imaging followed by narrow band imaging for detecting early neoplasia in Barrett's esophagus. *Gastrointest Endosc* 2006; **64**: 176–85.

15 Borovicka J, Fischer J, Neuweiler J *et al*. Autofluorescence endoscopy in surveillance of Barrett's esophagus: a multicenter randomized trial on diagnostic efficacy. *Endoscopy* 2006; **38**: 867–72.

16 Chak A, Wallace MB, Poneros JM. Optical coherence tomography of Barrett's esophagus. *Endoscopy* 2005; **37**: 587–90.

17 Li XD, Boppart SA, Van Dam J *et al*. Optical coherence tomography: advanced technology for the endoscopic imaging of Barrett's esophagus. *Endoscopy* 2000; **32**: 921–30.

18 Evans JA, Nishioka NS. The use of optical coherence tomography in screening and surveillance of Barrett's esophagus. *Clin Gastroenterol Hepatol* 2005; **3**: S8–S11.

19 Pfau PR, Sivak MV, Chak A *et al*. Criteria for the diagnosis of dysplasia by endoscopic optical coherence tomography. *Gastrointest Endosc* 2003; **59**: 196–202.

20 Isenberg G, Sivak MV, Chak A *et al*. Accuracy of endoscopic optical coherence tomography lin the detection of dysplasia in Barrett's esophagus: a prospective, double-blinded study. *Gastrointest Endosc* 2005; **62**: 825–31.

21 Paddock SW, Fellers TJ, Davidson MW. Introduction to confocal microscopy. *Microscopy U*. Nikon USA. February 17, 2006. <http://www.microscopyu.com/articles/confocal/confocalintrobasics.html>.

22 Hoffman A, Goetz M, Vieth M *et al*. Confocal laser endomicroscopy: technical status and current indications. *Endoscopy* 2006; **38**: 1275–83.

23 Wang TD. Confocal microscopy from the bench to the bedside. *Gastrointest Endosc* 2005; **62**: 696–7.

24 Kiesslich R, Gossner L, Goetz M *et al*. In vivo histology of Barrett's esophagus and associated neoplasia by confocal laser endomicroscopy. *Clin Gastroenterol Hepatol* 2006; **4**: 979–87.

25 Savoy AD, Wallace MB. EUS in the management of the patient with dysplasia in Barrett's esophagus. *J Clin Gastroenterol* 2005; **39**: 263–7.

26 Pech O, May A, Gunter E *et al*. The impact of endoscopic ultrasound and computed tomography on the TNM staging of early cancer in Barrett's esophagus. *Am J Gastroenterol* 2006; **101**: 2223–9.

27 Shami VM, Villaverde A, Stearns L *et al*. Clinical impact of conventional endosonography and endoscopic ultrasound-guided fine-needle aspiration in the assessment of patients with Barrett's esophagus and high-grade dysplasia or intramucosal carcinoma who have been referred for endoscopic ablation therapy. *Endoscopy* 2006; **38**: 157–61.

28 Waxman I, Raju GS, Critchlow J *et al*. High-frequency probe ultrasonography has limited accuracy for detecting invasive adenocarcinoma in patients with Barrett's esophagus and high-grade dysplasia or intramucosal carcinoma: a case series. *Am J Gastroenterol* 2006; **101**: 1773–9.

CHAPTER 5

EMR Techniques

LIEBWIN GOSSNER AND CHRISTIAN ELL

Summary

Endoscopic mucosal resection (EMR) has gained more and more importance in the treatment of early gastrointestinal neoplasia over the last few years. The choice of the different available techniques depends on the site, the macroscopic type of the tumor, and the personal experience of the endoscopist. The 'suck and cut' technique with ligation device or cap should be favored over normal strip biopsy in the upper gastrointestinal tract because of the larger size of the resected specimen and its technical feasibility.

EMR of gastrointestinal lesions is a safe and effective method but should only be performed by experienced endoscopists in high volume centers.

Introduction

The technique of endoscopic mucosal resection (EMR) emerged in the early 1970s. Since then EMR in the gastrointestinal (GI) tract has been used for many years as a diagnostic and therapeutic procedure for early malignancies. Initially intended to allow large biopsy, it actually became an alternative to surgery for the treatment of flat, sessile lesions, including high-grade intraepithelial neoplasia, carcinomas such as mucosal cancer, or superficial submucosal cancer (sm1) with a low risk of spread to lymph nodes. The technique is used especially in the east Asian region, and data concerning EMR for this indication are sparse in Western publications.

In a 1984 publication, Tada et al. [1] for the first time described the use of 'strip-off biopsy' as a treatment option in early gastric carcinoma. The first

Endoscopic Mucosal Resection. Edited by M. Conio, P. Siarsema, A. Repici and T. Ponchon. © 2008 Blackwell Publishing. ISBN 978-1-4051-5885-5.

EMR procedures for early esophageal carcinoma were carried out in the early 1990s, again by Japanese endoscopists [2]. It was only several years later that the first Western research groups published their experience in EMR for esophageal neoplasias [3,4]. This was the start of the triumphant progress of EMR as a therapeutic and diagnostic procedure in the upper and lower gastrointestinal tract. A large number of different EMR techniques was described (see Table 5.1). The original strip biopsy technique advocated by Tada involved only injection and snaring – a submucosal injection is used to form a bleb, which is then cut by snare strangulation. Hirao *et al.* [5] described a technique involving injection, pre-cutting, and snaring, in which after submucosal injection, the target mucosa is cut with an electrocautery needle-knife, and the isolated mucosa is then captured with a snare wire. Makuuchi [6] later developed an endoscopic esophageal mucosal resection (EEMR) tube method, with which a larger resected specimen can be obtained.

Our own group now has more than 10 years' experience in EMR treatment for malignant lesions in the upper gastrointestinal tract, with more than 1000 ER procedures. We believe that the method of endoscopic mucosal resection using a cap (EMR-C) or a ligation device (EMR-L) are the simplest techniques for carrying out mucosectomy in any part of the gastrointestinal tract.

Table 5.1 Classification of endoscopic mucosal resection techniques

I Without suction
1. Strip-off biopsy (injection and snaring) [1]
2. Lift and cut biopsy, double-snare polypectomy (grasping and snaring) [7,8]
3. ER-HSE: endoscopic resection with hypertonic saline-epinephrine solution (injection, precutting, and snaring) [5]
4. EMR-T: endoscopic mucosal resection using a transparent overtube (grasping and snaring using an overtube) [9]*

II With suction
1. EEMR: endoscopic esophageal mucosal resection, tube method (injection and snaring using an overtube) [6]
2. np-EEM: endoscopic esophageal mucosectomy under negative-pressure control (injection and snaring using an overtube) [10]
3. EMR-C: endoscopic mucosal resection using a transparent plastic cap (injection and snaring using a cap) [11]
4. EMR-L: endoscopic mucosal resection using a ligating device (endoscopic variceal ligation and snaring) [12]
5. Simple suction technique (snaring with a stiff snare) [4]

* These techniques are only available in the esophagus.

Principle

The organs of the GI tract basically consist of two major parts, the muscle layer and the mucosal layer. These two components are attached to each other by the loose connective tissue of the submucosa and can easily be separated. Thus, it is possible to resect the mucosa and submucosa without hurting the muscle layer. As the wall of the GI-tract is only about 4 mm thick, special management is required to avoid perforation. Correct lifting of the mucosa is therefore extremely important. Injecting saline or other liquids into the submucosal layer or mechanical lifting using special instruments, e.g. a ligation device are the easiest and most effective techniques for avoiding muscle involvement. After lifting the mucosa including the target lesion, it can be safely captured, grasped with the snare wire, and resected by electrocauterization.

Prior to EMR of gastrointestinal lesions, especially in the upper GI tract, a carefully done staging by experienced physicians including chromoendoscopy, endosonography with 7.5 MHz-probe and 20 MHz miniprobe, and computed tomography, abdominal ultrasound is crucial.

Different EMR techniques

Strip biopsy

Strip biopsy was first successfully used by Tada to treat early gastric carcinoma [1]. In this technique, a diathermy loop is introduced through the endoscope's working channel and positioned above a polypoid lesion. The lesion is caught by tightening the loop, and is slowly resected using electric cutting current. This technique can mainly be used in polypoid tumors (type I), as it is not possible to position the loop with flat lesions. Soehendra et al. [4] report successful ER treatment of two early squamous-cell carcinomas. No complications or recurrences were reported. Technically, ER was carried out using a monopolar diathermy–polypectomy loop, without prior injection under the lesion.

However, submucosal injection of a solution can also raise flat or depressed lesions (type II) so that they can be resected (the 'lift and cut' technique) – a method that was first described by Rosenberg in 1955 [13]. In addition to extending the range of target lesions in comparison with simple strip biopsy, this procedure also has other advantages. Injecting a solution of saline and epinephrine, for example, into the submucosa raises the early carcinoma, increasing the distance from the muscularis propria and thus reducing the risk of perforation. Since the wall of the entire gastrointestinal tract is only a few millimeters thick, this cushion is a very important safety factor. Another advantage of the injection technique is the reduced risk of hemorrhage due to the vasoconstriction produced by epinephrine and the compression caused by the injection itself.

The type of injection solution used has not been standardized. The solution most often used is saline with epinephrine or dextrose in various concentrations. We use 10 ml of a 1:100 000 epinephrine–saline solution. The advantage of the epinephrine solution, in comparison with the saline plus dextrose solution also used, is the vasoconstriction caused by the catecholamine and the resulting reduction in the risk of hemorrhage. A disadvantage of the epinephrine–saline mixture is its short disappearance time (3.0 min) in comparison with a 50% dextrose solution (4.7 min) and a 1% rooster comb hyaluronic acid solution (22.1 min). These data were obtained in an animal-experiment study in the porcine esophagus [14]. Hyaluronic acid therefore, is more frequently used for the submucosal injection. After placement of electro-markers, which mark the boundaries of the tumor with a sufficient safety margin, injection under the lesion with a mixture of hyaluronic acid, epinephrine, and indigo carmine follows.

Suck and cut technique

The 'suck-and-cut' technique is used in the esophagus more frequently than strip biopsy, due to the anatomical conditions, and is also the technique favored by our own group. With a simple strip biopsy, with or without mucosal injection, sufficiently large specimens cannot be obtained in the esophagus, particularly in flat neoplastic lesions. A study by Tanabe et al. [15] demonstrated that endoscopic suck-and-cut mucosectomy in early gastric cancer is more effective than strip biopsy with regard to the largest diameter of the resected specimen, the rate of en-bloc resection, and the complication rate.

In the early 1990s, Inoue and co-workers developed the cap technique, thereby improving the effectiveness of EMR in comparison with simple strip biopsy [16]. In the EMR cap technique (EMR-C), a specially developed transparent plastic cap is attached to the end of the endoscope. After injection under the target lesion, the lesion is sucked into the cap and resected with a diathermy loop that has previously been loaded onto a specially designed groove on the lower edge of the cap. Since injecting underneath early carcinomas often makes it difficult to distinguish them, prior marking of the lesion – e.g. using electrocautery – is recommended.

EMR with a ligation device (EMR-L) is another suction mucosectomy technique. In this method, the target lesion is sucked into the ligation cylinder, and a polyp is created by releasing a rubber band around it. The polyp is then resected at its base, either above or below the rubber band, using a diathermy loop (Fig. 5.1(a)–(e)). In this technique, the endoscope being used for resection

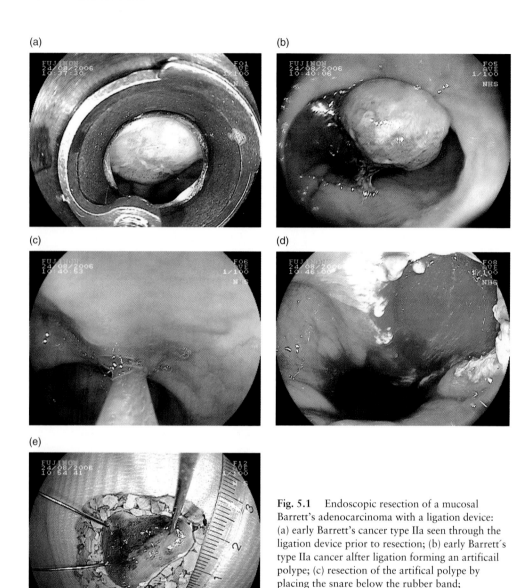

Fig. 5.1 Endoscopic resection of a mucosal Barrett's adenocarcinoma with a ligation device: (a) early Barrett's cancer type IIa seen through the ligation device prior to resection; (b) early Barrett's type IIa cancer alfter ligation forming an artificail polype; (c) resection of the artifical polype by placing the snare below the rubber band; (d) Resected area after EMR at the cardia: the muscular layer is clearly visible; (e) the resected specimen of 22 mm in diameter pinned on cork.

has to be withdrawn again and reintroduced in order to remove the ligation cylinder and introduce the loop. Ligation devices available include, in addition to single-use devices, a reusable ligator [17], with which comparable results can be achieved at reduced cost. The feasibility of this technique was demonstrated in patients with early Barrett's carcinoma and intraepithelial high-grade neoplasia and was presented by our own research group [18]. Complete remission was achieved in 82.5% of cases. Recent publications have also confirmed the effectiveness of EMR with the ligation technique in 50 patients with early neoplasia in short-segment Barrett's esophagus [19,20]. The intermediate results were similarly encouraging (average follow-up period 34 ± 10 months) in 115 patients treated [21].

A study published in 2003 by our research group compared the two suction mucosectomy techniques – the cap technique and the ligation technique – in the resection of early esophageal neoplasias [22]. In this prospective study, 100 consecutive endoscopic mucosal resections were performed in 70 patients with early esophageal cancer. Fifty resections were carried out with the ligation device without prior injection, and 50 resections using the cap technique with prior submucosal injection with a diluted epinephrine–saline solution. The main criteria were the maximum diameter of the resected specimen, the resection area, and the complication rate. No significant differences were observed between the two groups with regard to the maximum diameter of the resected specimens and the resection area after 24h. There was only a slight advantage for the ligation group in patients who had had prior treatment. One minor bleeding incident occurred in each group, but no severe complications were seen.

Furthermore, our own experience with EMR treatment in the suck and cut technique for early squamous-cell carcinoma in 39 patients has now for the first time in a Western country confirmed the promising data presented by Asian researchers [23,24]. Complete remission was achieved in 79% of cases; recurrences or metachronous carcinomas were observed in five. Complications encountered involved mild bleeding, not requiring transfusion, in 3% of cases (three of 94 resections). Similarly good results were presented by Narahara *et al.* [25]. In 21 patients, successful mucosectomy of a total of 25 mucosal carcinomas was carried out after injection of a saline solution under the lesion. None of the patients had experienced a recurrence after two years.

If the lesion is so large that it is not possible to remove it using a single 'suck-and-cut' EMR procedure, then it is also permissible even with malignant lesions to resect the entire lesion using the so-called 'piecemeal' method . The long-term results with this method are as good for early gastric cancer, for example, as with en-bloc resections [26]. Endoscopic submucosal dissection (ESD) might offer the chance of entire en-bloc resection of large lesions (see Chapter 11).

In addition to the suck-and-cut mucosectomy and strip biopsy techniques, EMR using a double-channel endoscope has also been reported by several research groups [27]. In this method, a grasping forceps is used to pull the target lesion through a diathermy loop that has been introduced through the second working channel. The lesion is then resected with the loop. Due to the large caliber of the endoscope required, double-channel procedures appear to be very difficult, especially at the esophagogastric junction, and may even be almost impossible in the inverted position in short-segment Barrett's neoplasia.

Risks and complications of EMR

ER involves certain risks, and should therefore only be carried out by experienced endoscopists. The most frequent complication of EMR is hemorrhage. Arterial bleeding is very rare. By contrast, oozing venous bleeding is not uncommon; it is usually not associated with a drop in hemoglobin, and is easily arrested by injection. Hemorrhage after EMR usually occurs during the first 12–24 h. For this reason, we regularly carry out check-up endoscopies after 24 h following EMR in the upper gastrointestinal tract, and only discharge patients when the findings are unremarkable.

By contrast, hemorrhage following EMR in the colon can appear up to 14 days after resection. According to a Japanese study, the risk of bleeding after ER in the colon is 1.15%, compared with 0.66% with simple polypectomy [28].

After circular ER in the esophagus, colon, or duodenum, scar formation and stenosis can develop during the subsequent months. However, this complication can be satisfactorily treated by bougienage or dilatation.

Perforation is the most serious complication of ER. Depending on the size and location of the lesion, the figures for the frequency of perforation in the upper gastrointestinal tract range from 0.06% to 5% [29]. Perforations in the stomach can usually by treated conservatively by closing the site with metal clips and administering antibiotic treatment and parenteral nutrition. The risk of perforation after ER in the colon is approximately 0.35% – much higher than with simple polypectomy (0.053%) [28].

In experienced hands, ER is a safe method of resecting dysplastic lesions and early carcinomas in the gastrointestinal tract, and it has decisive advantages over other local endoscopic treatment procedures (such as thermal destruction and photodynamic therapy): the histological processing of the resection specimen provides information about the depth of infiltration of the individual wall layers, and whether complete removal with healthy margins has been achieved. This means that even when a patient has an advanced carcinoma that has not been detected before treatment and which is not suitable for local endoscopic therapy, surgical resection can still be carried out.

References

1 Tada M, Murata M, Murakami F et al. Development of the strip-off biopsy [in Japanese]. Gastroenterol Endosc 1984; 26: 833–9.
2 Makuuchi H, Machimura T, Soh Y et al. Endoscopic mucosectomy for mucosal carcinomas in the esophagus. Jap J Surg Gastroenterol 1991; 24: 2599–603.
3 Inoue H, Endo M, Takeshita K et al. Endoscopic resection of carcinoma in situ of the esophagus accompanied by esophageal varices. Surg Endosc 1991; 5: 182–4.
4 Soehendra N, Binmoeller KF, Bohnacker S et al. Endoscopic snare mucosectomy in the esophagus without any additional equipment: a simple technique for resection of flat early cancer. Endoscopy 1997; 29: 380–3.

5 Hirao M, Masuda K, Asanuma T *et al.* Endoscopic resection of early gastric cancer and other tumors with local injection of hypertonic saline-epinephrine. *Gastrointest Endosc* 1988; **34:** 264–9.

6 Makuuchi H. Endoscopic mucosal resection for early esophageal cancer. *Dig Endosc* 1996; **8:** 175–9.

7 Takekoshi T, Baba Y, Ota H *et al.* Endoscopic resection of early gastric carcinomas: results of a retrospective analysis of 308 cases. *Endoscopy* 1994; **26:** 352–8.

8 Martin TR, Onstad GF, Silvis SE, Vennes JA. Lift and cut biopsy technique for submucosal samplings. *Gastrointest Endosc* 1976; **23:** 29–30.

9 Inoue H, Endo M. Endoscopic esophageal mucosal resection using a transparent tube. *Surg Endosc* 1990; **4:** 198–201.

10 Kawano T, Miyake S, Yasuno M. A new technique for endoscopic esophageal mucosectomy using a transparent overtube with intraluminal negative pressure (np-EEM). *Dig Endosc* 1991; **3:** 159–67.

11 Inoue H, Takeshita K, Hori H, Muraoka Y, Yoneshima H, Endo M. Endoscopic mucosal resection with a cap-fitted panendoscope for esophagus, stomach, and colon mucosal lesions. *Gastrointest Endosc* 1993; **39:** 58–62.

12 Fleischer DE, Wang GQ, Dawsey S *et al.* Tissue band ligation followed by snare resection (band and snare): a new technique for tissue acquisition in the eosphagus. *Gastrointest Endosc* 1996; **44:** 67–72.

13 Rosenberg N. Submucosal saline wheal as a safety factor in fulguration of rectal and sigmoid polyps. *Archives of Surgery* 1955; **70:** 120–3.

14 Conio M, Rajan E, Sorbi D, Norton I, Herman L, Filiberti R, Gostout CJ. Comparative performance in the porcine esophagus of different solutions used for submucosal injection. *Gastrointest Endosc* 2002; **56:** 513–16.

15 Tanabe S, Koizumi W, Kokutou M *et al.* Usefulness of endoscopic aspiration mucosectomy as compared with strip biopsy for the treatment of gastric mucosal cancer. *Gastrointest Endosc* 1999; **50:** 819–22.

16 Inoue H, Endo M. A new simplified technique of endoscopic esophageal mucosal resection using a cap-fitted panendoscope. *Surg Endosc* 1993; **6:** 264–5.

17 Ell C, May A, Wurster H. The first reusable multiple-band ligator for endoscopic hemostasis of variceal bleeding and mucosal resection. *Endoscopy* 1999; **31:** 738–40.

18 Ell C, May A, Gossner L *et al.* Endoscopic mucosal resection of early cancer and high-grade dysplasia in Barrett's esophagus. *Gastroenterology* 2000; **118:** 670–7.

19 May A, Gossner L, Pech O *et al.* Intraepithelial high-grade neoplasia and early adenocarcinoma in short-segment Barrett's esophagus (SSBE): curative treatment using local endoscopic treatment techniques. *Endoscopy* 2002; **34:** 604–10.

20 Behrens A, May A, Gossner L *et al.* Curative treatment for high-grade intraepithelial neoplasia in Barrett's esophagus. *Endoscopy* 2005; **37:** 999–1005.

21 May A, Gossner L, Pech O *et al.* Local endoscopic therapy for intraepithelial high-grade neoplasia and early adenocarcinoma in Barrett's oesophagus: acute-phase and intermediate results of a new treatment approach. *Eur Journal Gastroenterol Hepatol* 2002; **14:** 1085–91.

22 May A, Gossner L, Behrens A, Ell C. A prospective randomized trial of two different suck-and-cut mucosectomy techniques in 100 consecutive resections in patients with early cancer of the esophagus. *Gastrointest Endosc* 2003; **58:** 167–75.

23 Pech O, Gossner L, May A *et al.* Endoscopic resection of superficial esophageal squamous cell carcinomas: Western experience. *Am J Gastroenterol* 2004; **99:** 1226–32.

24 Pech O, May A, Gossner L *et al.* Curative endoscopic therapy in patients with early esophageal squamous-cell carcinoma or high-grade intraepithelial neoplasia. *Endoscopy* 2007; **39:** 30–5.

25 Narahara H, Iishi H, Tatsuta M *et al.* Effectiveness of endoscopic mucosal resection with submucosal saline injection technique for superficial squamous carcinomas of the esophagus. *Gastrointest Endosc* 2000; **52:** 730–4.

26 Tanabe S, Koizumi W, Mitomi H *et al.* Clinical outcome of endoscopic aspiration mucosectomy for early stage gastric cancer. *Gastrointest Endosc* 2002; **56:** 708–13.

27 Noda M, Kobayashi N, Kanemasa H *et al*. Endoscopic mucosal resection using a partial trans-
    parent hood for lesions located tangentially to the endoscope. *Gastrointest Endosc* 2000; **51:**
    338–43.
28 Okamoto H, Tanaka S, Haruma K *et al*. Japanese review of complications and measure by
    endoscopic treatment for colorectal tumor between 1989–1993 [in Japanese]. *Hiroshima
    Igaku (Journal of Hiroshima Medical Assocation)* 1996; **49:** 585–91.
29 Rembacken BJ, Gotoda D, Fuji T, Axon ATR. Endoscopic mucosal resection. *Endoscopy*
    2001; **33:** 709–18.

CHAPTER 6

Endoscopic Mucosal Resection in the Esophagus

MASSIMO CONIO

Introduction

Most gastrointestinal cancers are diagnosed at an advanced stage, with a poor survival rate despite treatment including major surgery and adjuvant therapy. Superficial cancers have a low risk of lymph node involvement, allowing effective local treatment.

Endoscopic mucosal resection (EMR), is a promising therapeutic option for removal of superficial gastrointestinal tract carcinomas (Table 6.1) [1].

Unlike ablative methods such as photodynamic therapy (PDT) and argon plasma coagulation (APC), EMR permits histologic assessment of the entire specimen.

Until 30 to 40 years ago, most esophageal cancers in developed countries were squamous-cell carcinomas (SCC). Since then, the proportion of esophageal adenocarcinomas (AC), related to gastroesophageal reflux and Barrett's esophagus (BE) has risen to constitute 46–50% of new cases of esophageal cancer [2]. BE is a complication of long-standing gastroesophageal reflux disease, which is present in about 5–10% of patients undergoing endoscopy for reflux symptoms.

Cancer can develop in patients with BE over several years, through a sequence encompassing non-dysplastic metaplasia, low-grade dysplasia (LGD), high-grade dysplasia (HGD), and invasive AC. HGD is found in fewer than 5% of patients with BE [3]. Pathological examination showed unrecognized cancers in 38–73% of patients who had surgery for HGD [4]. When HGD is diagnosed, slides should be reviewed by an expert pathologist because there is substantial variation within and between observers.

Endoscopic Mucosal Resection. Edited by M. Conio, P. Siersema, A. Repici and T. Ponchon. © 2008 Blackwell Publishing. ISBN 978-1-4051-5885-5.

Table 6.1 Considerations for endoscopic mucosal resection of a gastrointestinal lesion.

When EMR is suitable

• Patient with LGD, HGD, or IMC without lymph node involvement
• Lesion at risk for malignancy or progression
• Complete resection technically feasible

Favorable outcomes depend on

• Complete removal of the lesion
• Absence of synchronous lesions or invasive disease

EMR: endoscopic mucosal resection; HGD: high-grade dysplasia; IMC: intramucosal cancer; LGD: low-grade dysplasia.

Classification of early cancers

In the Vienna classification, gastrointestinal neoplastic lesions are defined as non-invasive or invasive. The non-invasive group includes LGD and HGD, where the basement membrane is not infiltrated. Invasive lesions include intramucosal cancers (IMC) and neoplasms infiltrating the submucosa [5].

Risk of lymph node metastases

To better define the risk for lymph node metastases, mucosal (m) and submucosal (sm) layers have each been divided in three sections: m1 (epithelium), m2 (lamina propria), m3 (muscularis mucosae) and sm1 (sm1a, b, c), sm2, and sm3. Nodal metastases were found in 0% of patients with m1 and m2 SCC of the esophagus, 4% with m3, and 26% with sm1 tumors.

The full thickness of the submucosa can be carefully evaluated in surgically resected specimens. This allows a semiquantitative measurement of the depth of the tumor invasion, and the fractioning of the submucosa in three equal layers. Buskens *et al.* [6] studied 77 esophagectomy specimens containing HGD or T1 carcinoma. Node metastases occurred with 23% sm2, and 69% sm3 tumors, but not in m1, m2, m3, and sm1 lesions. They concluded that m1, m2, m3, and sm1 lesions could be treated endoscopically if the lesion is <30 mm, well-differentiated, and without lymphangitic invasion. This detailed histologic analysis is not possible for specimens obtained with EMR, as it is difficult to entirely resect the submucosa.

The evaluation of EMR specimens can be carried out using a quantitative micrometric measure (μ) of the depth of the invasion, starting from the bottom of the mucosa. The risk of lymph node metastasis is related to a defined cutoff. In the squamocellular cancer (SCC) of the esophagus, when infiltration is

<200 μm the risk of nodal metastases is low. It increases to 36–47% with deeper invasion.

For BE, a submucosal infiltration of 500 μm has been proposed, as the risk of nodal metastases is low. However, a 20–25% risk of node involvement with submucosal infiltration has been reported [7,8].

Endoscopic mucosal resection techniques

Before performing EMR, in patients with visible mucosal abnormalities, the lesion margins should be identified, to avoid incomplete resection. Chromo-endoscopy with methylene blue, or Lugol iodine may show the extent of cancers. Marking the periphery of the lesion with electrocautery helps to determine the area of EMR.

The lesion can be removed 'en bloc', or 'piecemeal'. Piecemeal resection increases the complication rate, histologic assessment of the margins is diffi-cult, and the recurrence risk is higher. The maximum recommended diameter for 'en bloc' resection is 20 mm in the esophagus.

Submucosal injection

The gastrointestinal wall has two components, mucosal and muscle layers, attached by a loose connective tissue of submucosa. Injection of a fluid into the submucosa creates a cushion between the lesion and the deeper layers of the gut wall before removal.

Submucosal fluid injection facilitates EMR and avoids thermal damage to the muscularis propria, helping to identify invasive lesions, with sensitivity 100% and specificity 99%. If the lesion does not lift, EMR should not be attempted.

A more durable submucosal fluid cushion may result in safer procedures. Several solutions have been proposed, some of which have been tested only experimentally: normal saline with or without adrenaline, 50% dextrose, glyc-eol (10% glycerol and 5% fructose), hyaluronic acid, and hydroxypropyl methylcellulose.

The effects of hydroxypropyl methylcellulose were studied in the esophagus of pigs. The mean submucosal fluid cushion duration was 36 min. The authors stated that 0.83% hydroxypropyl methylcellulose was able to create a longer lasting submucosal esophageal cushion, without causing tissue reaction. The leakage of the solution from the needle puncture site was the main cause of short-lasting cushions [9].

In our endoscopic practice, we use normal saline plus adrenaline solution (1/100.000). A small amount of methylene blue is added to the solution to facilitate visibility in the esophageal wall. Whatever solution is used, it is necessary to avoid repeated needle injections so that the fluid is not dispersed.

Strip biopsy

Strip biopsy is the simplest technique as it requires the use of a polypectomy snare. After the submucosal injection, the open snare is placed around a portion of the lesion and gently pressed against the mucosa. Excess air has to be aspirated from the hollow organ to decrease distention and to allow an easy grasp of the targeted lesion. After snare excision, air is again insufflated to visualize the resected area and to allow the residual tissue to be removed. Resections have to be performed until complete removal of the lesion, and exposure of the muscularis propria. A barbed snare can be used to facilitate the grasping of the tissue.

The size of the samples obtained with this procedure ranges between 10 and 15 mm.

Soehendra *et al.* [10] reported the use of a monofilament stainless steel wire (0.4 mm) polypectomy snare to perform esophageal EMR, without submucosal injection.

Endoscopic mucosal resection 'cap-assisted' (EMR-C)

A transparent plastic cap is preloaded on the endoscope tip. Inside the cap is a gutter which positions the opened polypectomy snare. After submucosal injection, the cap is pressed against the mucosa, the lesion is aspirated into the cap, and resected (Fig. 6.1).

It has been reported that EMR-C is better and safer than standard snare resection. Experimental studies have corroborated this assertion, showing that EMR-C is safer and easier than snare resection. The diathermic injury is less marked, allowing a better histologic assessment of depth and margin involvement.

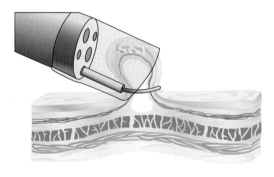

Fig. 6.1   EMR-C technique.

The major limitation of the EMR-C is that it is impossible to evaluate the amount of tissue that, after the suction, has been grasped with the polypectomy snare. An excessive suction could entrap the muscularis propria, causing a transmural resection. To decrease the risk of perforation it is advisable to sever the grasped tissue after having decreased the aspiration into the cap. This maneuver allows the muscularis propria to retract, returning to its original position.

In our experience results of EMR-C, in terms of width and depth of the resected specimen, are sometimes unpredictable in the lower esophagus, close to the esophagogastric junction. Sometimes, the diameter of the resection is no wider than 10 mm, and resection can involve fibers of the muscularis propria. Caution is advised when the EMR involves the esophagogastric junction. During the aspiration into the cap, a large amount of gastric tissue, which is softer and more mobile, may be captured by the snare or by the rubber, leading to potential complications.

'Suck and ligate' technique

EMR can be performed using a standard variceal ligator device. An artificial polyp is created and resection is performed with a polypectomy snare (Fig. 6.2). The diameter of the resected mucosa ranges between 10 and 15 mm [11–12].

When performing this technique, the submucosa injection is not always necessary, as the risk of damaging the muscularis propria is nil [13].

The ligation technique has proved to be more effective than EMR-C in treating recurrences in patients who previously underwent endoscopic treatments. The fibrosis of the scar did not impede placement of the rubber [14].

A randomized study showed no significant difference between the 'suck and ligate' technique, without submucosal injection, and EMR-C after injection for

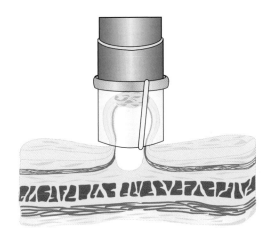

Fig. 6.2 'Suck and ligate' technique.

early esophageal AC or SCC. After EMR, 57% of patients had residual neoplasia at the first follow-up [14].

This method is cumbersome, requiring the repeated introduction of endoscopes. The first endoscope allows the submucosal injection, and the second instrument is placed into the esophagus to release the band. As a standard polypectomy snare cannot be introduced through the operative channel of the instrument, the endoscope is withdrawn and the first endoscope is reintroduced to resect the artificial polyp.

A novel multibanding mucosectomy device (MMD) (Duette®, Cook Ireland Ltd, Limerick, Ireland) has been recently presented (Fig. 6.3). It consists of a modified multi-band variceal ligator and a mini hexagonal polypectomy snare which can be passed through the ligator handle. The lesion is suctioned into the barrel of the ligator and a rubber band is placed on it creating a pseudopolyp. This pseudopolyp is resected using the preloaded snare.

The setup is similar to a standard multiple-band ligator device. Up to six resections per device may be made.

Complications

Despite the advantages of EMR compared to surgery, it must be remembered that it is an invasive technique and complications may occur. However, in the literature, deaths have not been reported. To minimize the risks, only experienced endoscopists should undertake EMR in an appropriate environment.

Early complications include bleeding and perforation. Bleeding has been reported in up to 14% of procedures. Usually it is intraprocedural, but it can occur later than 24 hours following EMR. Epinephrine and hemoclips are useful to control spurting hemorrhage. Bleeding was reported in 4–20% of esophageal

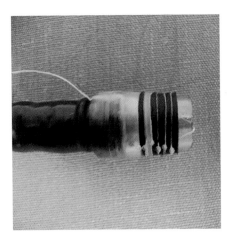

Fig. 6.3 Multibanding mucosectomy device (Duette®).

SCC, in about 10% of patients with lesions in BE, and in 12% of early gastric cancer (EGC) [15–18]. The perforation risk during EMR is 0.1–5% [19].

When EMR involves over three-quarters of the esophageal circumference, stenosis can occur a few weeks later. Mucosal defects longer than 3 cm were also associated with greater severity of the stenosis. This complication has been reported in up to 30% of cases [20–22]. A few sessions of endoscopic dilation can solve the stricture [23].

Indications for esophageal EMR are summarized in Table 6.2 and outcomes in Table 6.3.

Esophageal squamous-cell cancer

In Japan EMR is a common therapy for SCC confined within the lamina propria mucosae. EMR is also used for lesions infiltrating the muscularis mucosae, as the survival is comparable with esophagectomy [24]. Indications for EMR of SCC are listed in Table 6.2.

Table 6.2   Indications for esophageal EMR.

Benign epithelial lesions	Hyperplastic-adenomatous polyps
	Granular cell tumor
Early-stage AC	Well or moderately differentiated SCC–AC
	IIa, IIb, IIc <20 mm
	m1 or m2 cancers
Barrett's esophagus	HGD–IMC within visible mucosal abnormalities
	Circumferential EMR for endoscopically
	undetectable foci of HGD in SSBE*
	Visible areas of LGD to refine the histologic
	diagnosis

AC: adenocarcinoma; EMR: endoscopic mucosal resection; HGD: high-grade dysplasia; IMC: intramucosal cancer; LGD: low-grade dysplasia; SCC: squamous-cell cancer; SSBE: short-segment Barrett's esophagus.

Table 6.3   EMR outcome in esophageal lesions.

Complications	Resection rate (%)	Recurrence (%)	Surgery after EMR (%)
Squamous-cell cancer			
Bleeding: 4–20%	64–94	0–10	0–15
Perforation: 1–5%			
Barrett's esophagus			
Bleeding: 0–33%	60–95	0–31	0–15
Stenosis: 0–30%			

EMR: endoscopic mucosal resection.

Multicentric squamous epithelial dysplasia is common, and chromoendo-scopy with Lugol is useful in these patients. Lugol-voiding lesions (LVLs) have been observed in association with synchronous and metachronous multiple esophageal cancer in patients with head and neck cancer. It has been reported that patients with multiple LVLs are at risk of developing local recurrences after EMR [25]. Multiple synchronous lesions have been reported in 26–31% of patients with SCC. Metachronous lesions may also develop [26,27].

Local recurrence after EMR has been reported in 2.4–7.8%, and it has been associated with piecemeal resection [28]. After EMR in patients with superficial SCC, the five-year survival rate is up to 95% [29,30].

M1 and m2 SCC have little likelihood of lymph node metastasis [31]. EMR in 25 patients with superficial (m1) SCC showed no recurrence after a mean follow-up of two years [16].

It has been reported that patients with m3 areas attached or infiltrating the lamina muscularis mucosae showed lymph node or distal metastasis. These patients should be treated with curative surgery.

Few reports have analysed the outcome of EMR in patients with invasive cancer. Shimizu et al. compared 26 patients with SCC invading the muscularis mucosae or the submucosa, treated by EMR, with 44 comparable patients undergoing surgery. Survival was similar in the two groups, 77% vs. 84% [24]. A European group treated 39 SCC patients. Success was obtained in 79% of cases, and local recurrences or metachronous lesions occurred in five (13%). Bleeding (3%) was managed endoscopically. Two patients died because of disease progression [32].

A multimodality approach in patients with SCC invading the submucosa was tried in 18 patients. After EMR, chemo-radiotherapy was given if lymph node involvement was present or suspected. No local recurrences were observed [33].

Barrett's esophagus

Endoscopic therapy aims to remove the dysplastic BE, allowing restoration of squamous epithelium. Methods used to remove HGD include PDT and APC, as well as EMR (Table 6.4). After these procedures, patients need long-term control of acid reflux with proton pump inhibitors or antireflux surgery.

Patients with visible areas of LGD, should also undergo EMR. There are reports on the natural history of LGD, showing the progression to HGD and AC. Skacel et al. [34] followed 25 patients with LGD (mean follow-up: 26 months) and seven patients (28%) developed HGD, while AC occurred in two of them.

EMR could become a therapeutic alternative to surgical esophagectomy, which involves substantial morbidity, and a mortality rate of 3–5% [20,31].

Table 6.4 Therapeutic options for superficial cancer in Barrett's esophagus.

Treatment	Pros	Cons	Outcome
EMR	✓ Histologic assessment ✓ Removal of circumferential BE up to 4 cm	✓ Incomplete treatment of invisible foci of HGD	✓ Favorable in superficial cancer
PDT	✓ Easy to perform	✓ Lack of adequate histological examination ✓ Photosensitivity and esophageal stenosis	✓ Favorable in superficial cancer
Laser	✓ Deep penetration	✓ Lack of adequate histological examination ✓ Persistence of buried metaplastic epithelium	✓ Few data available
APC	✓ Non-contact technique ✓ Easy to perform	✓ Lack of adequate histological examination ✓ Persistence of buried metaplastic epithelium	✓ Few data available
Surgery	✓ Complete removal of BE ✓ Histological evaluation of lymph nodes	✓ Morbidity and mortality not negligible ✓ Worsening of quality of life	✓ Radical treatment

APC: argon plasma coagulation; BE: Barrett's esophagus; EMR: endoscopic mucosal resection; HGD: high-grade dysplasia; PDT: photodynamic therapy.

The review of 161 cases who underwent EMR showed a survival rate of 100%, and an overall recurrence rate ranging between 0% and 15.8% [35,36].

The frequency of synchronous cancers undetected by endoscopy and biopsy in patients with long segment of BE (LSBE) is about 50%.

EMR maximizes the histological assessment of the lesion, allowing definition of both its lateral extent and its depth. It changes the pathological stage in many patients. Ablative methods (PDT, APC) prevent any histopathological assessment. Histological reclassification has been reported in up to 75% of patients after EMR, because of biopsy sampling error and observer interpretation (Table 6.5). In a previous chapter of this book, the role of EUS as a staging tool has been discussed. However, several reports have demonstrated that EMR is more accurate than EUS in staging superficial esophageal tumors.

In our experience, we observed a change in histological diagnosis in 26% of patients with BE who underwent EMR [37]. Mino-Kenudson *et al.* [38] also reported a change in the histologic diagnosis in 37% of the cases.

When HGD is found in short BE tongues (≤30 mm) EMR can remove all the metaplastic epithelium.

The sequential use of EMR to remove the visible areas of HGD, followed by PDT for invisible foci of malignant disease has been proposed in patients with LSBE. Buttar *et al.* [22] successfully treated 17 non-surgical patients who had superficial esophageal cancer. EMR improved staging in 47% of cases. Stenosis after PDT was recorded in 30% of patients.

After PDT, microscopic remnants of specialized intestinal metaplasia ('buried Barrett') can persist under the neosquamous epithelium, making an adequate endoscopic follow-up even more difficult [39]. It has also been shown that genetic abnormalities persist in the residual BE after PDT treatment.

At present, the majority of articles have reported the endoscopic resection of nodular lesions, or mucosal abnormalities, easily detectable at endoscopy.

Circumferential mucosectomy is an attractive option as it would permit the complete removal of the metaplastic epithelium, with an optimal histologic assessment, avoiding the persistence of buried remnants of BE (Figs 6.4(a)–(c)).

Our group was the first to demonstrate the feasibility of circumferential mucosectomy in an animal model [40].

Circumferential EMR was performed in 12 patients with non-visible HGD and/or IMC. The authors removed 30–40 mm in length and three-quarters of the circumference in each session, using a polypectomy snare without submucosal injection. Two strictures were resolved with bougienage. No recurrences were observed during a median nine-month follow-up [21].

In another study, circumferential EMR was carried out in 21 patients with HGD or mucosal cancer. Three patients had residual disease: one underwent surgery, and two, treated with chemo-radiotherapy, were free of disease after

Table 6.5 Selected studies on EMR in high-grade dysplasia or early cancer in Barrett's esophagus.

Author	Patients (n)	Size of lesion cm (mean)	Histology pre-EMR	Histology post-EMR	Complications	Surgery	Follow-up months (mean)	Recurrence
Peters et al., 2006 [42]	33	Median 1.5	9 HGD 10 HGD/AC 14 AC	22 HGD 8 EC 3 no dysplasia	Bleeding: 45% (15/33) Stenosis: 3% (1/33)	5	Median 19	15% (5/33)
Mino-Kenudson et al., 2005 [38]	18	1.1	10 HGD 7 IMC 2 AC	2 LGD 5 HGD 10 IMC 2 AC	0	1 (AC)	ND	5% (9/19)
Conio et al., 2005 [37]	39	1.5	35 HGD 4 IMC	5 LGD 27 HGD 2 IMC 5 SMC	Bleeding: 10% (4/39) Stenosis: 3% (1/39)	3 (AC)	Median 35	
Giovannini et al., 2004 [41]	21	1.6	12 IMC 9 AC	12 HGD 9 AC	Bleeding: 19%	1	18	0

Continued

Table 6.5 (Continued)

Author	Patients (n)	Size of lesion cm (mean)	Histology pre-EMR	Histology post-EMR	Complications	Surgery	Follow-up months (mean)	Recurrence
Seewald et al., 2003 [21]	12	ND	3 HGD 2 HGD/IMC 7 IMC	2 BE 1 LGD 5 HGD 4 AC	Bleeding: 33% (4/12) Stenosis:17% (2/12)	0	Median 9	0
May et al., 2002 [20]	80	ND	7 HGD 73 EC	11/80 AC	Bleeding: 6% Stenosis: 4%	0	34	30% (24/80)
Buttar et al., 2001 [22]	17	ND	7 IMC 10 AC	7 IMC 10 AC	Bleeding: 6% (1/17) Stenosis: 0	1	13	0
Nijhawan et al., 2000 [36]	25	ND	2 BE 8 LGD 5 HGD 9 AC 1 other	2 BE 3 LGD 5 HGD 13 AC 2 other	0	2/13 (AC)	14.6	31% (4/13 AC)
Ell et al., 2000 [35]	35	0.9	3 HGD 32 EC	3 HGD 32 EC	Bleeding: 20% (7/35)	ND	12	11% (4/35)

AC: invasive adenocarcinoma; BE: Barrett's esophagus; EC: early cancer; EMR: endoscopic mucosal resection; HGD: high-grade dysplasia; IMC: intramucosal cancer; LGD: low-grade dysplasia; ND: not detectable.

(a)   (b)

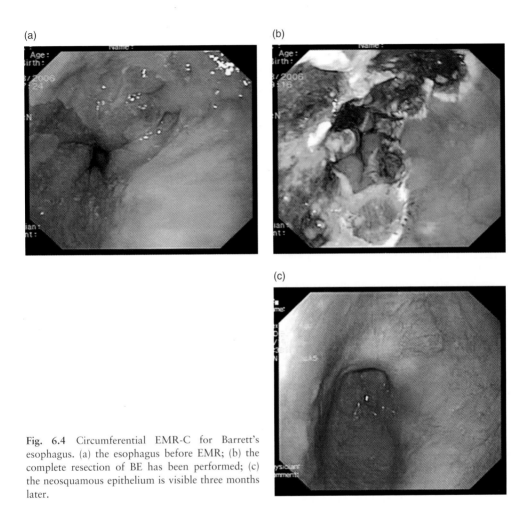

(c)

Fig. 6.4 Circumferential EMR-C for Barrett's
esophagus. (a) the esophagus before EMR; (b) the
complete resection of BE has been performed; (c)
the neosquamous epithelium is visible three months
later.

18 and 24 months, respectively. Two local recurrences were retreated by EMR.
Neosquamous epithelium was observed in 75% of patients [41].

Stepwise radical endoscopic resection has been performed in 37 patients, with
a median BE length of 4 cm (range 3–5 cm). APC was used in 34 patients to
complete the resection. Complete eradication was achieved in all 37 patients,
and no recurrences were detected during a median follow-up of 11 months.
The overall complication rate was 2%. One patient suffered esophageal perforation, which was managed conservatively by placing a suction tube and a
duodenal feeding tube [42].

Soehendra et al. [43] performed MMD–EMR in ten patients with BE containing HGD and/or IMC. No submucosal injection was performed. In five out
of ten patients with circumferential BE (median length: 4 cm; range: 2–9 cm)

complete EMR was performed in one session. Four patients required more sessions (median: three). One patient underwent surgery due to the multifocality of HGD and/or IMC. No immediate complications occurred. Seven patients developed strictures that were managed successfully by weekly bougienage (median sessions: five). The authors conclude that MMD–EMR is safe, but it is associated with a high stricture rate if circumferential EMR is performed in one session.

After the EMR, a double dose of proton pump inhibitors must be given to these patients. The acid suppressive therapy should be started one week before the endoscopic procedure. The anacid environment favors the regrowth of squamous mucosa.

Conclusions

EMR represents an important advance in endoscopic therapy, making it possible to remove early cancers from the esophagus. Randomized control studies comparing EMR with surgery are still lacking. However, the quality of life after EMR is undoubtedly better than after esophagectomy.

Patients need careful evaluation prior to EMR, and only those with superficial lesions and no lymph node involvement should undergo the procedure. EMR is less invasive than surgical resection, and thus morbidity and mortality are lower. Compared to PDT and APC, EMR can more easily remove full thickness mucosa without damaging the underlying muscle and permits histologic evaluation of all the resected mucosa. Improved endoscopic equipment would allow circumferential EMR to be performed as a unique treatment, without other mucosal ablative procedures.

The 'suck and ligate' technique, now performed with the Duette® device, can be more reassuring for endoscopists undertaking this endotherapy technique. However, more data are necessary to establish the safety and effectiveness of this procedure.

Surveillance after EMR is mandatory to detect recurrences at an early stage, which could be easily retreated with EMR. In patients who underwent EMR for SCC, chromoendoscopy with Lugol should be performed. According to the literature and our experience, we would suggest performing endoscopic follow-up one month after EMR, then every three months for the first year, and every six months thereafter.

More training, and exposure, is required for gastroenterologists and trainees to become conversant with this technique. EMR should be performed by competent endoscopists, able to cope with procedural complications. However, more data are needed on the long-term results.

References

1 Conio M, Ponchon T, Blanchi S, Filiberti R. Endoscopic mucosal resection. *Am J Gastroenterol* 2006; **101**: 653–6.

2 Brown LM, Devesa SS. Epidemiologic trends in esophageal and gastric cancer in the United States. *Surg Oncol Clin N Amer* 2002; **11**: 235–56.

3 Gopal DV, Lieberman DA, Magaret N *et al.* Risk factors for dysplasia in patients with Barrett's esophagus: results from a multicenter consortium. *Dig Dis Sci* 2003; **48**: 1537–41.

4 Conio M, Cameron AJ, Chak A, Blanchi S, Filiberti R. Endoscopic treatment of high-grade dysplasia and early cancer in Barrett's esophagus. *Lancet Oncol* 2005; **6**: 311–21.

5 Willis J, Riddell RH. Biology versus terminology: East meets West in surgical pathology. *Gastrointest Endosc* 2003; **57**: 369–76.

6 Buskens CJ, Westerterp M, Lagarde SM *et al.* Prediction of appropriateness of local endoscopic treatment for high-grade dysplasia and early adenocarcinoma by EUS and histopathologic features. *Gastrointest Endosc* 2004; **60**: 703–10.

7 Nigro JJ, Hagen JA, DeMeester TR *et al.* Prevalence and location of nodal metastases in distal esophageal adenocarcinoma confined to the wall: implications for therapy. *J Thorac Cardiovasc Surg* 1999; **117**: 16–23.

8 Stein HJ, Feith M, Mueller J, Werner M, Siewert JR. Limited resection for early adenocarcinoma in Barrett's esophagus. *Ann Surg* 2000; **232**: 733–42.

9 Feitoza AB, Gostout CJ, Burgart LJ, Burkert A, Herman LJ, Rajan E. Hydroxypropyl methylcellulose: a better submucosal fluid cushion for endoscopic mucosal resection. *Gastrointest Endosc* 2003; **57**: 41–7.

10 Soehendra N, Binmoeller KF, Bohnacker S *et al.* Endoscopic snare mucosectomy in the esophagus without any additional equipment: a simple technique for resection of flat early cancer. *Endoscopy* 1997; **29**: 380–3.

11 Suzuki H. Endoscopic mucosal resection using ligating device for early gastric cancer. *Gastrointest Endosc Clin N Am* 2001; **11**: 511–18.

12 Suzuki Y, Hiraishi H, Kanke K *et al.* Treatment of gastric tumors by endoscopic mucosal resection with a ligating device. *Gastrointest Endosc* 1999; **49**: 192–9.

13 Fleischer DE, Wang GQ, Dawsey S *et al.* Tissue band ligation followed by snare resection (band and snare): a new technique for tissue acquisition in the esophagus. *Gastrointest Endosc* 1996; **44**: 68–72.

14 May A, Gossner L, Behrens A *et al.* A prospective randomized trial of two different endoscopic resection techniques for early stage cancer of the esophagus. *Gastrointest Endosc* 2003; **58**: 167–75.

15 Overholt BF, Panjehpour M, Haydek JM. Photodynamic therapy for Barrett's esophagus: follow-up in 100 patients. *Gastrointest Endosc* 1999; **49**: 1–7.

16 Narahara H, Iishi H, Tatsuda M *et al.* Effectiveness of endoscopic mucosal resection with submucosal saline injection technique for superficial squamous carcinomas of the esophagus. *Gastrointest Endosc* 2000; **52**: 730–4.

17 Tani M, Takeshita K, Saeki I *et al.* Protection of residue or recurrence following endoscopic mucosal resection for gastric tumours lesion [Japanese]. *Progress Digest Endosc* 1997; **50**: 74–8.

18 Chonan A, Mochizuki F, Ando M *et al.* Endoscopic mucosal resection (EMR) of early gastric cancer: usefulness of aspiration EMR using a cap-fitted scope. *Dig Endosc* 1998; **10**: 31–6.

19 Tani M, Sakai P, Kondo H. Endoscopic mucosal resection of superficial cancer in the stomach using the cap technique. *Endoscopy* 2003; **35**: 348–55.

20 May A, Gossner L, Pech O *et al.* Local endoscopic therapy for intraepithelial high-grade neoplasia and early adenocarcinoma in Barrett's oesophagus: acute-phase and intermediate results of a new treatment approach. *Eur J Gastroenterol Hepatol* 2002; **14**: 1085–91.

21 Seewald S, Akaraviputh T, Seitz U *et al.* Circumferential EMR and complete removal of Barrett's epithelium: a new approach to management of Barrett's esophagus containing high-grade intraepithelial neoplasia and intramucosal carcinoma. *Gastrointest Endosc* 2003; **57**: 854–9.

22 Buttar NS, Wang KK, Lutzke LS, Krishnadath KK, Anderson MA. Combined endoscopic mucosal resection and photodynamic therapy for esophageal neoplasia within Barrett's esophagus. *Gastrointest Endosc* 2001; **54**: 682–8.

23 Katada C, Muto M, Manabe T, Boku N, Ohtsu A, Yoshida S. Esophageal stenosis after endoscopic mucosal resection of superficial esophageal lesions. *Gastrointest Endosc* 2003; **57**: 165–9.

24 Shimizu Y, Tsukagoshi H, Fujita M, Mosokawa M, Kato M, Asaka M. Long-term outcome after endoscopic mucosal resection in patients with esophageal squamous cell carcinoma invading the muscularis mucosae or deeper. *Gastrointest Endosc* 2002; **56**: 387–90.

25 Katada C, Muto M, Manabe T, Ohtsu A, Yoshida S. Local recurrence of squamous-cell carcinoma of the esophagus after EMR. *Gastrointest Endosc* 2005; **61**: 219–25.

26 Pesko P, Rakic S, Milicevic M, Bulajic P, Gerzic Z. Prevalence and clinicopathologic features of multiple squamous cell carcinoma of the esophagus. *Cancer* 1994 ; **73**: 2687–90.

27 Kuwano H, Ohno S, Matsuda H, Mori M, Sugimachi K. Serial histologic evaluation of multiple primary squamous cell carcinomas of the esophagus. *Cancer* 1988; **61**: 1635–8.

28 Nomura T, Boku N, Ohtus A *et al.* Recurrence after endoscopic mucosal resection for superficial esophageal cancer. *Endoscopy* 2000; **32**: 277–80.

29 Takeshita K, Tani M, Inoue H *et al.* Endoscopic treatment of early esophageal or gastric cancer. *Gut* 1997; **40**: 123–7.

30 Inoue H. Endoscopic mucosal resection for esophageal and gastric mucosal cancers. *Can J Gastroenterol* 1998; **12**: 355–9.

31 Kodama M, Kakegawa T. Treatment of superficial cancer of the esophagus: a summary of responses to a questionnaire on superficial cancer of the esophagus in Japan. *Surgery* 1998; **123**: 432–9.

32 Pech O, Gossner L, May A, Vieth M, Stolte M, Ell C. Endoscopic resection of superficial esophageal squamous-cell carcinomas: Western experience. *Am J Gastroenterol* 2004; **99**: 1226–32.

33 Ota M, Ide H, Hayashi K *et al.* Multimodality treatments with endoscopic mucosal resection of esophageal squamous cell carcinoma with submucosal invasion. *Surg Endosc* 2003; **17**: 1429–33.

34 Skacel M., Petras RE, Gramlich TL, Sigel JE, Richter JE, Goldblum JR. The diagnosis of low-grade dysplasia in Barrett's esophagus and its implications for disease progression. *Am J Gastroenterol* 95: 3383–7.

35 Ell C, May A, Gossner L *et al.* Endoscopic mucosal resection of early cancer and high-grade dysplasia in Barrett's esophagus. *Gastroenterology* 2000; **118**: 670–7.

36 Nijhawan PK, Wang KK. Endoscopic mucosal resection for lesions with endoscopic features suggestive of malignancy and high-grade dysplasia within Barrett's esophagus. *Gastrointest Endosc* 2000; **52**: 328–32.

37 Conio M, Repici A, Cestari R *et al.* Endoscopic mucosal resection for high-grade dysplasia and intramucosal carcinoma in Barrett's esophagus: an Italian experience. *World J Gastroenterol* 2005; **11**: 6650–5.

38 Mino-Kenudson M, Bruge WR, Puricelli WP *et al.* Management of superficial Barrett's epithelium-related neoplasms by endoscopic mucosal resection: clinicopathologic analysis of 27 cases. *Am J Surg Pathol* 2005; **29**: 680–6.

39 Overholt BF, Panjehpour M, Halberg DL. Photodynamic therapy for Barrett's esophagus with dysplasia and/or early stage carcinoma: long-term results. *Gastrointest Endosc* 2003; **58**: 183–8.

40 Conio M, Sorbi D, Batts KP, Gostout CJ. Endoscopic circumferential esophageal mucosectomy in a porcine model: an assessment of technical feasibility, safety, and outcome. *Endoscopy* 2001; **33**: 791–4.

41 Giovannini M, Bories E, Pesenti C *et al.* Circumferential endoscopic mucosal resection in Barrett's esophagus with high-grade intraepithelial neoplasia or mucosal cancer. Preliminary results in 21 patients. *Endoscopy* 2004; **36**: 782–7.

42 Peters FP, Kara MA, Rosmolen WD *et al.* Stepwise radical endoscopic resection is effective for complete removal of Barrett's esophagus with early neoplasia: a prospective study. *Am J Gastroenterol* 2006; **101**: 1449–57.

43 Soehendra N, Seewald S, Groth S *et al.* Use of modified multiband ligator facilitates circumferential EMR in Barrett's esophagus. *Gastrointest Endosc* 2006; **63**: 847–52.

CHAPTER 7

Stomach

NAOMI KAKUSHIMA, MITSUHIRO FUJISHIRO, AND
TAKUJI GOTODA

Introduction

Application of endoscopic resection (ER) to early gastric cancer (EGC) is limited
to lesions with no risk of nodal metastasis. In Japan, many methods of ER have
been developed and become popular, probably due to the high incidence of
gastric cancer and the fact that more than half of Japanese patients with gastric
cancer are diagnosed at an early stage. Empirical indications for endoscopic
mucosal resection (EMR) have been considered as differentiated type mucosal
cancers without ulcerative findings, 2 cm in size if elevated or 1 cm if depressed
or flat. This indication was widely accepted for a long time because of two
aspects. First, these lesions have no risk of nodal metastasis; second, the size and
shape of these lesions are resectable in a single fragment, by the conventional
ER technique of EMR. Recently, remarkable technical advances and acquisition
of data about lesions with no risk of nodal metastasis brought us to a new gen-
eration of ER – the development of endoscopic submucosal dissection (ESD)
and expanding the indication for EGC. In this chapter the indication, techniques and outcomes of various EMR and ESD methods are described.

Expanding indication for endoscopic resection

EGC is defined to a mucosal or submucosal invasive cancer (T1 cancer)
irrespective of the presence of nodal metastasis. Lesions indicated for ER
should be EGC with no risk of nodal metastasis and ability to be resected in a
single fragment. Using a large database of more than 5000 patients with EGC
who underwent gastrectomy with D2 lymph node dissection, a criteria of node
negative tumors has been defined (Table 7.1)[1]. For the lesions described
in Table 7.1, gastrectomy with lymph node dissection would be excessive

Endoscopic Mucosal Resection. Edited by M. Conio, P. Siersema, A. Repici and
T. Ponchon. © 2008 Blackwell Publishing. ISBN 978-1-4051-5885-5.

Table 7.1 Early gastric cancer with no risk of nodal metastasis.

Expanded criteria for endoscopic mucosal resection	Incidence (no. with metastasis/ total number)	95% confidence interval
Intramucosal cancer Differentiated adenocarcinoma, no lymphatic vessel invasion, irrespective of ulcer findings, tumor ≤3 cm	0/1230	0–0.3
Intramucosal cancer Differentiated adenocarcinoma, no lymphatic vessel invasion, without ulcer findings, irrespective of tumor size	0/929	0–0.4
Intramucosal cancer Undifferentiated adenocarcinoma, no lymphatic vessel invasion, without ulcer findings, tumor ≤2 cm	0/141	0–2.6
Cancer with minute submucosal penetration (≤500 μm) Differentiated adenocarcinoma, no lymphatic vessel invasion, irrespective of ulcer findings, tumor ≤3 cm	0/145	0–2.5

treatment if en bloc resection were possible by ER, and would impair the quality of life afterwards. At present, lesions with preoperative endoscopic diagnosis of differentiated-type intramucosal cancer without ulcer findings, or differentiated-type intramucosal cancer no larger than 3 cm in diameter with ulcer findings, are considered as expanding the indication for ER. Because the margins of undifferentiated-type cancer lesions are often difficult to delineate, and because preoperative diagnosis of minute submucosal invasive cancer is difficult, ER for these lesions should be carefully considered.

Conventional ER methods are technically limited by lesions greater than 2 cm in diameter and by lesions with ulcer findings in respect of en bloc resection. Until the development of ESD, the approach to those lesions was only by piecemeal technique. Visual inspection of the resected site following piecemeal resection is often difficult, particularly if bleeding occurs, which may result in incomplete tumor removal. In addition, it is difficult to achieve a thorough pathologic evaluation from fragmented specimens after piecemeal resection. To facilitate reconstruction after piecemeal resection, and to confirm the completeness of the resection of the entire lesion, marking around the lesion before resection is useful. However, piecemeal resection has been associated with an increased recurrence rate and the inability to assess the specimen fully, which gives rise to uncertainty about the treatment's efficacy [2]. Therefore, for lesions larger than 2 cm in diameter and lesions with ulcer findings, ESD ensures more complete and efficient removal of the tumor in a single fragment.

Techniques and history of EMR

Just cut, or lift and cut technique

Simple polypectomy was first described in Japan in 1968. Protruded tumors with a stalk can be easily resected by polypectomy. For resection of lesions without stalks, endoscopic double-snare polypectomy (EDSP) was devised by Takekoshi in 1988 [3]. EDSP consists of two procedures using a double-channel endoscope; a sessile or depressed lesion is transformed into a subpedunculated shape by being pulled upward by one snare, and then another snare catching the pseudostalk and excising the lesion with high frequency electric current (HFEC).

Inject, lift and cut technique

From the early 1980s to the 1990s, methods using injection solution before resection were reported, including the strip biopsy method by Tada in 1984 [4], and four-point fixation endoscopic mucosal resection by Inatsuchi and colleagues [5].

Strip Biopsy Method. After marking around the lesion with the tip of a standard needle knife, saline with diluted epinephrine (1:100 000) is injected into the submucosal layer under the lesion with an injection needle. A double-channel endoscope is required, and both a snare and a pair of grasping forceps are advanced through the working channels. The forceps are passed through the opened snare to grasp the lesion, and gently pulled back through the opened snare. When the lesion is completely pulled into the snare, the snare is closed and the lesion is resected with HFEC. Small lesions without ulcer findings regardless of shape can be resected with this method, but the location applicable is limited.

Inject, suck and cut technique

In the early 1990s, several EMR techniques using a single-channel endoscope were reported. These techniques are characterized by using suction to capture the lesion. EMR with cap (EMRC) [6], endoscopic aspiration mucosectomy (EAM) [7], and EMR with ligation (EMRL) [8] fall in this group. These techniques are applied to small lesions without ulcer findings regardless of shape, and to lesions located in narrow or angulated areas. They are popular both in Japan and in Western countries for their convenience.

EMRC method. A single-channel endoscope with a transparent cap fitted to the tip is used. After marking and injection as described before, a crescent-shaped snare (SD-221L-25; Olympus Co., Tokyo, Japan) is pre-looped into the groove of the rim of the cap. Pre-looping could be done by suctioning the normal mucosa with the cap, together with light pressing of the opened snare to rest along the inside groove of the cap. The lesion is then sucked into the cap, the snare is pushed down onto the base of the aspirated lesion and closed. The suction is released to determine whether the center of the lesion is captured into the snare. The lesion is removed by HFEC and aspirated within the cap. Different-sized caps are available according to the diameter of the endoscope and the size of the target lesion.

EAM method. After marking and injection, an aspiration mucosector (Top Co. Ltd, Tokyo, Japan) is attached to the tip of a single-channel endoscope. The lesion is aspirated into the mucosector and a snare is opened to catch the lesion. The lesion is removed by HFEC.

The major difference between EMRC and EAM is that the snare is advanced through the working channel in EMRC, whereas in EAM, it is advanced through an outer sheath, which is preset to the endoscope.

EMRL method. After marking, the endoscope is withdrawn to fit a variceal ligation device (MD-48809, Sumitomo Bakelite Co., Tokyo, Japan). After submucosal injection, the lesion is ligated by the rubber band and snared below the rubber band.

The techniques given above are generally known as conventional ER/EMR methods (Figs 7.1(a)–(d)) compared to the following method. Conventional methods are safe, easy and convenient to use for small lesions. For lesions larger than 20 mm in diameter piecemeal resection is frequently performed using these methods because of technical limitations. To overcome technical problems of en bloc resection using conventional EMR methods, the following method has recently been developed.

Endoscopic submucosal dissection (ESD)

Inject, mucosal incision and submucosal dissection technique

The concept of this method was first reported by Hirao and colleagues in 1988 [9], and was named endoscopic resection with hypertonic saline–epinephrine solution (ERHSE). In this technique, after injection of hypertonic saline and diluted epinephrine, the periphery of the lesion was cut using a needle knife, followed by snaring. However, it has not been popular due to its difficulty and high complication rates.

It became common around 2000, with amelioration of the technique and development of numerous endoscopic equipments. At present, ESD with an

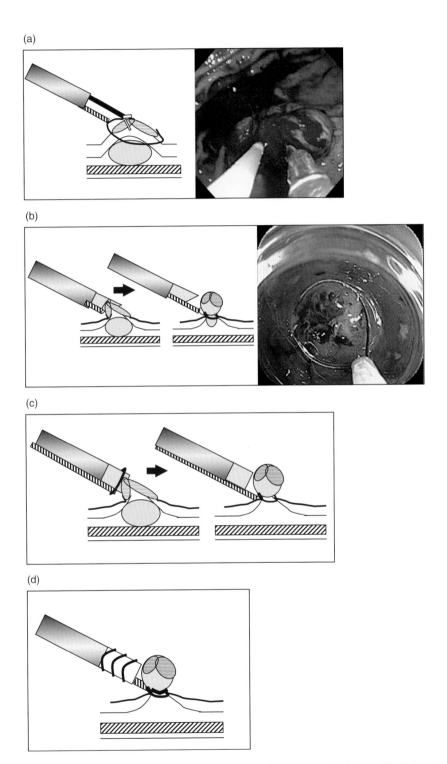

Fig. 7.1 Scheme of conventional endoscopic resection techniques. (a) Strip biopsy; (b) EMR with cap (EMRC); (c) Endoscopic aspiration mucosectomy (EAM); (d) EMR with ligation (EMRL).

insulation-tipped diathermic knife (IT-ESD) [10], EMR with sodium hyaluro-nate (EMRSH) [11], ER with a hook knife [12], ESD with the tip of an electro-surgical snare (thin type)/a flex knife [13], ER with a triangle-tipped knife by Inoue and colleagues [14], ER with a flush knife by Toyonaga and colleagues [15], and ER with a mucosectome by Kawahara and colleagues [16], have been developed to fall into this group, which is the latest category of ER, known as ESD. ESD requires special electrosurgical knives with an HFEC generator with an automatically controlled system (Endocut mode, Erbotom ICC200, ICC350, VIO300D, ERBE, Tubingen, Germany).

ESD is characterized by three steps – injecting fluid into the submucosa to elevate the lesion from the muscle layer; circumferential cutting of the sur-rounding mucosa of the lesion; and subsequent dissection of the connective tis-sue of the submucosa beneath the lesion (Fig. 7.2). It is controversial whether ESD should be included in EMR methods, or whether it is an independent ER technique. Most endoscopists in Japan now consider it as a novel and indepen-dent technique, because available outcomes are extremely different from those of conventional EMR methods.

ESD with IT-knife. Marking is made around the lesion with a needle knife. (forced coagulation 20W for ICC 200, swift coagulation 20 W, effect 4 for VIO300D). After injection with saline plus diluted epinephrine and indigo car-mine to raise the submucosal layer, a small initial incision is made by a needle knife (Endocut mode 80W, effect 3 for ICC 200, EndocutQ mode, duration 4, interval 1, effect 1 for VIO300D). The tip of the IT-knife is inserted from the ini-tial incision into the submucosal layer. Circumferential mucosal cutting outside the marking is performed by an IT-knife (Endocut mode 80 W, effect 3 for ICC200, EndocutQ mode, duration 4, interval 1, effect 1 or dry cut mode 50W, effect 4 for VIO300D). The ceramic ball prevents perforation of the knife. After completion of circumferential mucosal cutting, submucosal injection is added. Then, the submucosal layer under the lesion is directly dissected by the IT-knife until removal of the lesion.

ESD with Flex-knife. Marking is made around the lesion with the tip of a Flex-knife (soft coagulation mode 50 W for ICC 200, soft coagulation mode 50W, effect 5 for VIO300D). Injection is made with a glycerin solution (Glyceol™, a 10% glycerin with 0.9% NaCl plus 5% fructose solution, Chugai Pharmaceutical Co., Tokyo, Japan) with diluted epinephrine and indigo carmine. For lesions with ulcer findings, 1% 1900 kDa hyaluronic acid preparation is mixed to Glyceol with a ratio of 1:7 to achieve higher and long-lasting submucosal elevation. This special mixture of injection solution was developed through animal models and human studies considering the viscosity, tissue damage effect and lesion-lifting properties of several solutions [17–20]. Mucosal cutting (Endocut mode, 80W, effect 3 for ICC200, EndocutI mode, duration 4, interval 3, effect 3 for VIO300D)

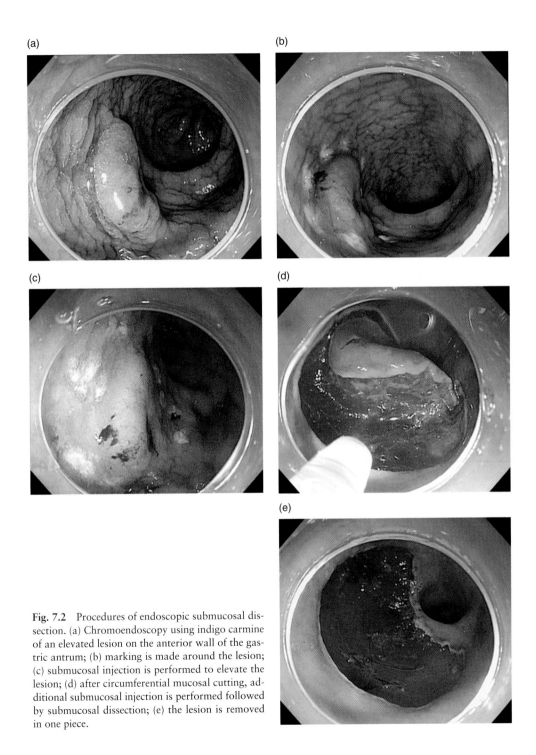

Fig. 7.2 Procedures of endoscopic submucosal dissection. (a) Chromoendoscopy using indigo carmine of an elevated lesion on the anterior wall of the gastric antrum; (b) marking is made around the lesion; (c) submucosal injection is performed to elevate the lesion; (d) after circumferential mucosal cutting, additional submucosal injection is performed followed by submucosal dissection; (e) the lesion is removed in one piece.

and submucosal dissection (forced coagulation mode 40W for ICC200, swift coagulation mode 40W, effect 4 for VIO300D) is performed step by step with the Flex-knife. A transparent attachment to the endoscope is frequently used during submucosal dissection, to achieve better vision and to get under the lesion into the submucosa.

The major advantages of ESD in comparison to other EMR methods are (a) the resected size and shape can be controlled, (b) en bloc resection is possible even for large lesions and difficult locations, and (c) lesions with ulcer findings are also resectable. Thus, ESD has rapidly become popular in Japan, and is applied to large lesions, ulcerative non-lifting lesions, lesions of the esophago-gastric junction [21] and recurrent lesions after previous endoscopic treatment [22]. Its efficacy and safety have also been reported in elderly patients [23]. The disadvantages of ESD are (a) it is time consuming, (b) the high complication rate of bleeding and perforation, and (c) technical difficulty. Available electrosurgical knives and other instruments for each method are provided in Table 7.2 and Fig. 7.3. Various knives and injection solutions have been

Table 7.2 Various instruments used in endoscopic submucosal dissection methods.

Method	Electrosurgical devices	Recommended injection solutions	Other instruments
IT-ESD	Insulation-tipped diathermic knife (IT knife, KD-610L, Olympus) Needle knife (KD-1L-1, Olympus)	Saline + diluted epinephrine	
ESD-flex knife	Flex knife (KD-630L, Olympus)	Glyceol* + diluted epinephrine ± hyaluronic acid	Transparent hood (D-201, Olympus)
ESD-hook knife	Hook knife (KD-620LR, Olympus) Needle knife (KD-1L-1, Olympus)	Glyceol* + diluted epinephrine	Transparent hood (D-201, Olympus)
EMRSH	Needle knife (KD-1L-1, Olympus)	Saline + diluted epinephrine + hyaluronic acid	Small caliber tip transparent (ST) hood (DH-15GR, 15CR, Fujinon Toshiba ES systems)

*Glyceol: a 10% glycerin with 0.9% NaCl plus 5% fructose solution (Glyceol™, Chugai Pharmaceutical Co., Tokyo, Japan).

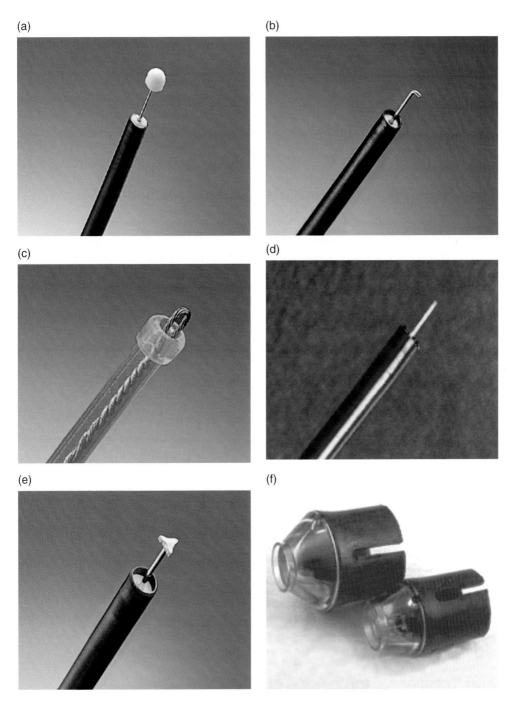

Fig. 7.3 Electrosurgical knives used in endoscopic submucosal dissection (ESD). (a) Insulation-tipped diathermic knife (IT-knife); (b) hook-knife; (c) flex-knife; (d) needle knife; (e) triangle-tipped knife (TT-knife); (f) small caliber tip transparent (ST) hood.

developed to lower the high complication rate and technical difficulty compared to EMR. Each ESD method has now achieved excellent outcomes, but they require highly skilled endoscopists, and a suitable training program is needed for this technique to become more widespread. Trainees in ESD should have skills of routine endoscopy and colonoscopy, target biopsy, endoscopic hemostasis techniques and a knowledge of simple EMR techniques. A trainee would gain early proficiency in ESD after 30 cases under the supervision of a mentor [24,25].

Pathological evaluation of the removed specimen

Whether a lesion may be included in the criteria of node-negative tumor is considered before treatment. However, at present, it is impossible to make a definite diagnosis of a tumor regarding depth, histological type and lymphatic vessel invasion before treatment. Therefore, a precise pathological evaluation of the resected specimen is essential, and an en bloc resection of the lesion is desirable in this respect.

After removal, the specimen should be oriented immediately before it is immersed in formalin. Orientation of the specimen is accomplished by fixing the periphery with thin needles on a plate of rubber or wood. The submucosal side of the specimen is faced to the plate. After fixation, the specimen is sectioned serially at 2 mm intervals parallel to a line that includes the closest part between the margin of the specimen and of the tumor, so that both lateral and vertical margins are assessed. The depth of tumor invasion is then evaluated microscopically along with the degree of differentiation and lymphatic or vascular involvement, if any.

After thorough pathological assessment, if the lesion is resected en bloc with negative margins of tumor, and if it fulfills the criteria for node-negative tumors, the treatment is judged as curative resection. For lesions with piecemeal resection but which are being judged as node-negative tumors, or lesions with histologically non-evaluable areas due to artifact or tissue burning, a periodical endoscopic follow-up should be performed to detect residual tumor or local recurrence. On the other hand, for lesions that do not fulfill the criteria of node-negative tumors, additional gastrectomy with nodal dissection should be strongly recommended.

Outcomes of EMR and ESD

The en bloc resection rate and local recurrence of ER reported before and after 2000 are described in Table 7.3. For lesions larger than 20 mm, the en

Table 7.3 Outcomes of various endoscopic resection methods before and after 2000.

Author	Methods	En bloc resection rate (%)			Local recurrence rate (%)
		≤10 mm	11–20 mm	≥21 mm	
Results before 2000					
Tada, 1998	Strip biopsy	70 (421/599)		–	11 (63/599)
Inatsuchi, 1996	Four-point fixation EMR	71 (30/42)	72 (21/29)	14 (2/14)	–
Takeshita, 1998	EMR-C	80 (44/55)	42 (24/57)	0 (0/9)	1.7 (2/118)
Torii, 1999	EAM	84 (52/62)		–	4.8 (3/62)
Hirao, 1998	ERHSE	63 (123/196)	44 (60/136)	19 (7/37)	2.3 (8/349)

		En bloc resection rate (%)		
		≤20 mm	>21 mm	
Recent results of ESD				
Ishigooka 2004	s-ERHSE	–	79 (36/46)	0 (0/46)
Hamanaka, 2004	IT-ESD	98 (455/463)	96 (235/245)	
Yahagi, 2004	ESD-thin type snare/flex knife	95 (56/59)		
Yamamoto, 2002	EMRSH	100 (37/37)	97 (32/33)	1 (1/70)
Oyama, 2004	ESD-hook knife	98 (202/207)	95 (103/109)	

EAM: endoscopic aspiration mucosectomy; EMR: endoscopic mucosal resection; EMR-C: EMR with cup; EMRSH: EMR with sodium hyaluronate; ERHSE: endoscopic resection with hypertonic saline-epinephrine solution; ESD: endoscopic submucosal dissection; IT-ESD: with insulation – tipped diathermic knife.

bloc resection rate is extremely low among conventional EMR methods, and local recurrence rates are around 10%. Although ESD was considered as a difficult and complicated technique when it was first described, after maturity of the techniques of ESD, en bloc resection rates became greater than 90%, regardless of size, and local recurrence rates became almost zero [26].

Complications of EMR include pain, bleeding, perforation, and stricture. Pain after EMR is mild. Complications of bleeding and perforation among

Table 7.4 Bleeding and perforation rate of various endoscopic resection methods.

Author	Method	Total cases	Bleeding (%)	Perforation (%)
EMR				
Torii, 1995	EAM	24	8.3	4
Tada, 1998	Strip biopsy	599	1.3	0.2
Chonan, 1998	EMR-C/ strip biopsy	123	7	4
Takeshita, 1998	EMR-C	121	14.9	0
Tanabe, 2002	EAM	206	13	1.5
Ohkuwa, 2001	Strip biopsy	88	4	1
Ono, 2001	Strip biopsy/ (IT-ESD)	479	–	5
ESD				
Hirao, 1996	ERHSE	373	6.7	2.9
Ohkuwa, 2001	IT-ESD	41	22	5
Yamamoto, 2002	EMRSH	70	4	0
Miyamoto, 2002	IT-ESD	123	38	0
Yahagi, 2004	Thin-type snare(flex-knife)	59	1.7	3.4
Oda, 2005	IT-ESD	1033	6	4

EAM: endosopic aspiration mucosectomy; EMR-C: endoscopic mucosal resection with cup; EMRSH: endoscopic musocal resection with sodium hyaluronate; ERHSE: endoscopic resection with hypertonic saline-epinephrine solution; IT-ESD: endoscopic submucosal dissection with insulation-tipped diathermic knife.

various EMR methods are described in Table 7.4. To prevent post-procedural bleeding, hemostasis of appearing vessels on the artificial ulcer after removing the specimen is essential. Hemostasis is performed by hemostatic forceps (HDB2422/HDB2418, Pentax), coagrasper (FD-410LR, Olympus), hot biopsy forceps, argon plasma coagulation or endoclips. With regard to perforation, recent case series suggest that small perforations immediately recognized can be successfully sealed with endoclips and treated conservatively by nasogastric suction, fasting and antibiotics, without emergency laparotomy [27].

Managements after EMR and ESD

Proton pump inhibitors (PPI) are administered to the patients to prevent postoperative bleeding and promote ulcer healing. Recent studies show that the duration of PPI treatment should be at least one week after EMR [28]. Large ulcers after ESD are reported to heal within 8 weeks after resection under antacid treatment [29].

Long-term outcomes after EMR

Long-term outcomes after EMR for small differentiated mucosal EGC less than 20 mm in diameter have been reported as comparable to those after gastrectomy. The disease-specific 5- and 10- year survival rates were 99% and 99% [30]. Long-term outcomes after ESD for lesions within the expanded indication are currently under investigation. On the other hand, endoscopic surveillance should be carried out in patients after EMR not only to detect local recurrence but also to detect metachronous gastric cancer (MGC). A recent study showed that the average time to detect a first MGC was 3.1 ± 1.7 years after EMR, and the cumulative three-year incidence was 5.9% [31]. In order to detect MGC at an early stage to perform a successful ER, an annual endoscopic surveillance program may be practical for post-ER patients.

Future perspectives

The advancement of technology in ESD is promising for further application in cancer treatment including esophageal and colorectal lesions. En bloc retrieval of lesions is essential for detailed histopathologic studies, which form the basis for stratification of treatment outcomes and patients' prognosis. ESD theoretically offers greater histopathological accuracy than conventional EMR methods or piecemeal resection. Although ESD developed at first as a subgroup of EMR, it is an innovative technique that can be applied to any mucosal lesions regardless of size and location, and which is expected to replace surgery. For less invasive surgery, ESD plus laparoscopic regional lymph node dissection has been investigated by Abe and colleagues [32]. Endoscopic full-thickness resection (EFTR) is under development in animal studies, to achieve more complete histological examination of the cancer by Ikeda and colleagues [33]. The field of ER is rapidly progressing, and in the near future, we will be able to completely avoid unnecessary gastrectomy.

References

1 Gotoda T, Yanagisawa A, Sasako M *et al.* Incidence of lymph node metastasis from early gastric cancer: estimation with a large number of cases at two large centers. *Gastric Cancer* 2000; **3**: 219–25.
2 Eguchi T, Gotoda T, Oda I *et al.* Is endoscopic one-piece mucosal resection essential for early gastric cancer? *Dig Endosc* 2003; **15**: 113–16.
3 Takekoshi T, Fujii A, Takagi K *et al.* The indication for endoscopic double snare polypectomy of gastric lesions (in Japanese with English abstract). *Stomach Intest* 1988; **23**: 387–98.
4 Tada M, Shimada M, Murakami F *et al.* Development of the strip-off biopsy (in Japanese with English abstract). *Gastroenterol Endosc* 1984; **26**: 833–9.

5 Tanaka M, Inatsuchi S. A four-point fixation method for the resection of early gastric cancer, with particular reference to the analysis of cases of incomplete resection. *Surg Endosc* 1997; **11**: 295–8.

6 Inoue H, Takeshita K, Hori H *et al.* Endoscopic mucosal resection with a cap-fitted panendoscope for esophagus, stomach, and colon mucosal lesion. *Gastrointest Endosc* 1993; **39**: 58–62.

7 Torii A, Sakai M, Kajiyama T *et al.* Endoscopic aspiration mucosectomy as curative endoscopic surgery; analysis of 24 cases of early gastric cancer. *Gastrointest Endosc* 1995; **42**: 475–9.

8 Masuda K, Fujisaki J, Suzuki H *et al.* Endoscopic mucosal resection using ligating device (EMRL) [in Japanese]. *Dig Endosc* 1993; **5**: 1215–19.

9 Hirao M, Masuda K, Asanuma T *et al.* Endoscopic resection of early gastric cancer and other tumors with local injection of hypertonic saline-epinephrine. *Gastrointest Endosc* 1988; **34**: 264–9.

10 Ohkuwa M, Hosokawa K, Boku N *et al.* New endoscopic treatment for intramucosal tumors using an insulated-tip diathermic knife. *Endoscopy* 2001; **33**: 221–6.

11 Yamamoto H, Yube T, Isoda N *et al.* A novel method of endoscopic mucosal resection using sodium hyaluronate. *Gastrointest Endosc* 1999; **50**: 251–6.

12 Oyama T, Tomori A, Hotta K *et al.* Endoscopic submucosal dissection of early esophageal cancer. *Clin Gastroenterol Hepatol* 2005; **3**: S67–70.

13 Yahagi N, Fujishiro M, Kakushima N *et al.* Endoscopic submucosal dissection for early gastric cancer using the tip of an electrosurgical snare (thin type). *Dig Endosc* 2004; **16**: 34–8.

14 Inoue H, Kudo S. A novel procedure of en bloc EMR using triangle-tipped knife (abstract). *Gastrointest Endosc* 2003; **57**: 494.

15 Toyonaga T, Nishino E, Hirooka T *et al.* Use of short needle knife for esophageal endoscopic submucosal dissection. *Dig Endosc* 2005; **17**: 246–52.

16 Kawahara Y, Imagawa A, Takenaka R *et al.* Improved endoscopic submucosal dissection (ESD) using a new device (mucosectome) (abstract). *Endoscopy* 2005; **37**: A20.

17 Fujishiro M, Yahagi N, Kashimura K *et al.* Different mixtures of sodium hyaluronate and their ability to create submucosal fluid cushions for endoscopic mucosal resection. *Endoscopy* 2004; **36**(7): 584–9.

18 Fujishiro M, Yahagi N, Kashimura K *et al.* Comparison of various submucosal injection solutions for maintaining mucosal elevation during endoscopic mucosal resection. *Endoscopy* 2004; **36**(7): 579–83.

19 Fujishiro M, Yahagi N, Kashimura K *et al.* Tissue damage of different submucosal injection solutions for EMR. *Gastrointest Endosc* 2005; **62**: 933–42.

20 Fujishiro M, Yahagi N, Nakamura M *et al.* Successful outcomes of a novel endoscopic treatment for GI tumors: endoscopic submucosal dissection with a mixture of high-molecular-weight hyaluronic acid, glycerin, and sugar. *Gastrointest Endosc* 2006; **63**: 243–9.

21 Kakushima N, Yahagi N, Fujishiro M *et al.* Efficacy and safety of endoscopic submucosal dissection for tumors of the esophagogastric junction. *Endoscopy* 2006; **38**: 170–4.

22 Yokoi C, Gotoda T, Hamanaka H *et al.* Endoscopic submucosal dissection allows curative resection of locally recurrent early gastric cancer after prior endoscopic mucosal resection. *Gastrointest Endosc* 2006; **64**: 212–18.

23 Kakushima N, Fujishiro M, Kodashima S *et al.* Technical feasibility of endoscopic submucosal dissection for gastric neoplasms in the elderly Japanese population. *J Gastroenterol Hepatol* (doi:10.1111/j.1440-1746.2006.04563.x, e-journal ahead of print).

24 Gotoda T, Friedland S, Hamanaka H *et al.* A learning curve for advanced endoscopic resection. *Gastrointest Endosc* 2005; **62**: 866–7.

25 Kakushima N, Fujishiro M, Kodashima S *et al.* A learning curve of endoscopic submucosal dissection for gastric epithelial neoplasms. *Endoscopy* (in press).

26 Oda I, Gotoda T, Hamanaka H *et al.* Endoscopic submucosal dissection for early gastric cancer: technical feasibility, operation time and complications from a large consecutive series. *Dig Endosc* 2005; **17**: 54–8.

27 Minami S, Gotoda T, Ono H *et al.* Complete endoscopic closure using endoclips for gastric perforation during endoscopic resection for early gastric cancer can avoid emergent surgery. *Gastrointest Endosc* 2006; **63**: 596–601.

28 Lee SY, Kim JJ, Lee JH *et al.* Healing rate of EMR-induced ulcer in relation to the duration of treatment with omeprazole. *Gastrointest Endosc* 2004; **60**: 213–17.

29 Kakushima N, Yahagi N, Fujishiro *et al.* The healing process of gastric artificial ulcers after endoscopic submucosal dissection. *Dig Endosc* 2004; **16**: 327–31.

30 Uedo N, Iishi H, Tatsuta M *et al.* Longterm outcomes after endoscopic mucosal resection for early gastric cancer. *Gastric Cancer* 2006; **9**: 88–92.

31 Nakajima T, Oda I, Gotoda T *et al.* Metachronous gastric cancers after endoscopic resection: how effective is annual endoscopic surveillance? *Gastric Cancer* 2006; **9**: 93–8.

32 Abe N, Mori T, Izumisato Y *et al.* Successful treatment of an undifferentiated early gastric cancer by combined en bloc EMR and laparoscopic regional lymphadenectomy. *Gastrointest Endosc* 2003; **57**: 972–5.

33 Ikeda K, Mosse A, Park P *et al,* Endoscopic full-thickness resection: circumferential cutting method. *Gastrointest Endosc* 2006; **64**: 82–9.

34 Ida K, Katoh T, Nakajima T *et al.* Outcome after using EMR according to standard guidelines for endoscopic treatment of early gastric cancer. *Stomach and Intestine* (in Japanese with english abstract) 2002; **37**: 1137–43.

35 Tanabe S, Koizumi W, Mitomi H *et al.* Clinical outcome of endoscopic aspiration mucosectomy for early stage gastric cancer. *Gastrointest Endosc* 2002; **56**: 708–13.

36 Ono H, Kondo H, Gotoda T *et al.* Endoscopic mucosal resection for treatment of early gastric cancer. *Gut* 2001; **48**: 225–9.

37 Yamamoto H, Kawata H, Sunada K *et al.* Success rate of curative endoscopic mucosal resection with circumferential mucosal incision assisted by submucosal injection of sodium hyalyronate. *Gastrointest Endosc* 2002; **56**: 507–12.

38 Miyamoto S, Muto M, Hamamoto Y *et al.* A new technique for endoscopic mucosal resection with an insulated-tip electrosurgical knife improves the completeness of resection of intramucosal gastric neoplasms. *Gastrointest Endosc* 2002; **55**: 576–81.

CHAPTER 8

Endoscopic Resection of Ampullary Neoplasms

GUIDO COSTAMAGNA AND CHRISTOPHER GOSTOUT

Introduction

Tumors of the ampulla of Vater are rare, accounting for less than 5% of all gastrointestinal tumors. Both benign (adenoma, hemangioma, leiomyoma, lipoma, and neurogenic tumors) and malignant tumors (adenocarcinoma, carcinoid tumors, signet-ring cell tumors, and choriocarcinoma) are well described. The most common lesions are tubulovillous adenomas and adenocarcinoma [1–3]. Although benign, ampullary adenomas have the potential to undergo malignant transformation, similar to the adenoma-carcinoma sequence in the colon and elsewhere in the gastrointestinal (GI) tract [4,5]. Ampullary adenomas may occur sporadically or in association with familial polyposis syndromes such as familial adenomatous polyposis (FAP) (Fig. 8.1). Such patients have a lifetime risk of up to 90% of developing ampullary and periampullary tumors [6,7]. Periampullary lesions involve the papilla and extend onto the surrounding duodenum to within 2 cm of the papilla (Fig. 8.2). Both ampullary and periampullary lesions are commonly grouped together and most often referred to as ampullary adenomas, as in this chapter [8]. The excision of adenomatous ampullary lesions is considered to prevent the eventual development of adenocarcinoma.

Benign ampullary lesions may be treated by surgical transduodenal ampullectomy. This involves complete en bloc excision of the ampulla of Vater together with a portion of healthy periampullary duodenal mucosa. The common bile duct and main pancreatic duct are then reinserted into the duodenal wall by two separate anastomoses. Pancreaticoduodenectomy (so-called Whipple's procedure or pylorus-preserving pancreaticoduodenectomy) remains the most commonly performed surgical procedure for large lesions, lesions with high grade dysplasia, and invasive neoplasms. However, pancreatic surgery is associated with increased morbidity and reported mortality rates between 1% and 9%, even in referral centers [7,9–15].

Endoscopic Mucosal Resection. Edited by M. Conio, P. Siersema, A. Repici and T. Ponchon. © 2008 Blackwell Publishing. ISBN 978-1-4051-5885-5.

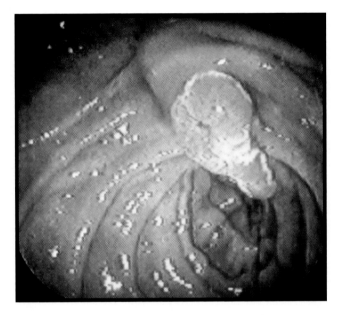

Fig. 8.1   Small ampullary adenoma in an FAP patient with classic distal 'goatee' extension inferiorly.

Endoscopic resection offers non-invasive management of benign ampullary neoplastic lesions. It is technically similar to polypectomy or mucosectomy, and involves excision (en bloc or piecemeal) of the Papilla of Vater which includes the overlying mucosa and submucosa of the ampulla of Vater, together with part of the sphincter of Oddi and the distal common bile duct and main pancreatic duct. Endoscopic snare resection is limited by the extent of tumor invasion into the bile or pancreatic ducts, or infiltration into the duodenal wall. Because of the low cost, minimal or no hospitalization, lack of a need for general anesthesia and low morbidity, endoscopic snare resection is advocated as first-line treatment for the management of benign, non-invasive ampullary neoplasms. However, despite widespread use in clinical practice, the indications, technique, and limitations of endoscopic resection vary between centers [16].

Indications for endoscopic snare resection

Over the past decade, there have been several retrospective reports on the technique of endoscopic snare resection with few published, prospective, randomized controlled studies [17]. For this reason, variations exist, even among experts, both for endoscopic technique and indications [3,18–28]. Endoscopic resection may be considered an alternative to surgical excision in patients with benign ampullary tumors, whereas invasive lesions should always be treated by surgical excision, unless short-term palliation for advanced malignancies is

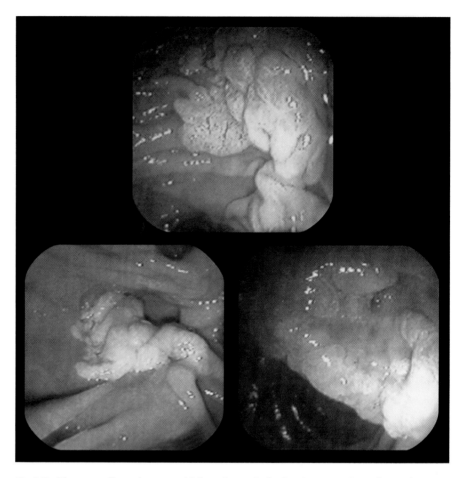

Fig. 8.2 Three ampullary adenomas with lateral spread of polyp tissue – 'periampullary' adenomas.

intended. Endoscopic resection may be considered to be curative if histological examination of the resected specimen shows the excision margins to be free of tumor and without any evidence of invasive carcinoma [29]. The morphologic characteristics of an ampullary lesion may be helpful in predicting whether the lesion is likely to be malignant or benign. The majority of ampullary and peri-ampullary tumors are diagnosed when they are advanced lesions. An attempt at endoscopic resection should, therefore, only be considered for small (e.g. ≤2 cm) or early lesions without evidence of deep invasion or tumor infiltration (Fig. 8.3). Submucosal invasion is associated with a high risk of lymph node metastases, and in such cases, endoscopic resection should not be attempted [12,30,31]. Published surgical studies reporting on the risk of lymph node metastasis associated with ampullary lesions, grouped together adenomatous lesions with in situ carcinoma, intramucosal carcinoma, and carcinoma with

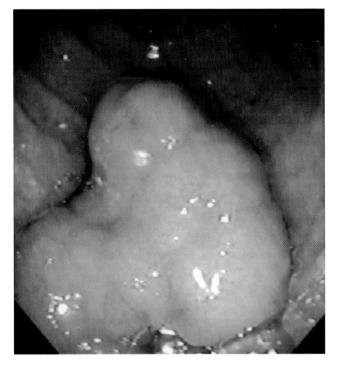

Fig. 8.3 Larger advanced ampullary adenoma which approaches the upper limit of size (2 cm) amenable to safe and complete endoscopic excision.

submucosal invasion as T1 lesions. For tumors limited to the ampulla of Vater (T1 according to the TNM classification), the rate of lymph node metastasis is reported to be between 0% and 22% [2,9,12,30,31]. Adenomas (low- and high-grade dysplasia) and carcinomas limited to the epithelium (in situ carcinoma) have a low risk of lymph node metastasis [32]. Lamina propria invasion (intramucosal carcinoma) is considered by some authors to be invasive carcinoma due to the rich mucosal lymphatic network in the ampullary area [33,34]. However, there is only scanty data on this particular issue in the scientific literature [16]. In general, submucosal invasion is considered to be a relative contra-indication to endoscopic resection [35], however, in patients with multiple comorbidities who are unfit for surgery, and those with very small, well-differentiated adenocarcinomas or small neuroendocrine tumors, endoscopic resection may be appropriate [30,36].

Indications for endoscopic resection in patients with FAP

In patients with FAP, endoscopic resection is controversial. Patients with FAP have a lifelong risk of developing periampullary adenomas necessitating regular, lifelong, endoscopic follow-up [6,37]. Patients with FAP have a high rate of recurrence following endoscopic resection. Ampullary adenomas in FAP progress slowly and may not become malignant [38–42]. Local recurrence following endoscopic resection is reported to be higher for lesions associated with familial polyposis syndromes as opposed to sporadic lesions [22]. For this reason, a less invasive approach has been considered by some authors for the endoscopic management of ampullary adenomas in FAP. Lifelong surveillance of the ampullary area can be facilitated after snare resection. Some authors advocate performing endoscopic papillectomy only in patients with adenomas showing high-grade dysplasia or in situ carcinoma, and repeated endoscopic surveillance and biopsy for the vast majority of patients [43].

Pre-operative staging: diagnosis of ampullary tumors and criteria for identifying invasive lesions

Duodenoscopy and ERCP

Ampullary neoplasms are readily diagnosed during ERCP. The macroscopic appearance of the papilla of Vater at duodenoscopy may predict whether the lesion is invasive or non-invasive. Macroscopic features suggesting malignancy include mucosal ulceration, spontaneous bleeding, induration or friability, and ill-defined or infiltrating margins [20,25]. In addition, the presence of duodenal infiltration can be assessed by grasping the base of the lesion with a snare and moving it back and forth. Lesions which are mobile are likely to be superficial and confined to the mucosal layer of the duodenum. Some authors consider the size of the lesion to be important when deciding whether to perform endoscopic resection [20,23,24]. Large lesions may be resected depending on the experience and expertise of the endoscopist.

In some cases, when the adenoma arises from the intra-ampullary epithelium, the whole papilla and overlying duodenal hood may be enlarged and bulging or protruding. The ERCP may identify extension of the neoplasm into the biliary or pancreatic duct prohibiting complete endoscopic excision (Fig. 8.4). In other cases, the ampullary lesion has a polypoid appearance without invasion into the bile- and pancreatic-ducts. In such cases, endoscopic resection is not technically difficult, even with large neoplastic lesions, which can require a piecemeal excision.

In early cases, the adenoma arises from the intestinal-type mucosa involving the papilla of Vater. Papillary adenomas occurring in patients affected by FAP belong to this specific group of lesions. In such cases, the adenoma tends to spread inferiorly, in a 'goatee' distribution and in time, laterally along the duodenal mucosa. Endoscopic resection in these presentations will additionally

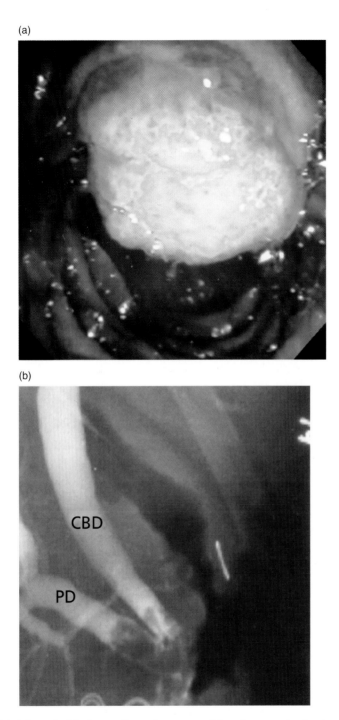

Fig 8.4 (a) A large 'bulging' ampullary adenoma suspicious for extensive involvement of the actual ampulla; (b) ERCP demonstrates actual invasion of the adenoma into both the common bile duct (CBD) and the pancreatic duct (PD). (c) EUS demonstrating the same extension of the adenoma into the CBD and PD.

(c)

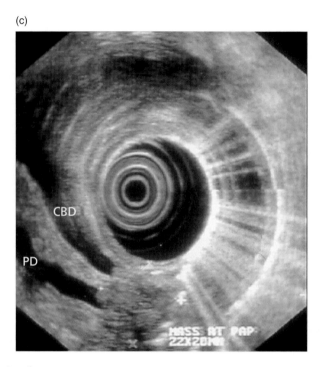

Fig 8.4   Continued

require piecemeal mucosectomy of the periampullary tissues as well as supplemental argon plasma coagulation of residual tissues for complete eradication of the lesion. Large lesions in excess of 2 cm are technically more difficult to resect. The risk of malignant transformation increases with the size of the lesion. Some authors advocate endoscopic resection for lesions with intraductal extension of up to 1 cm, in patients who are unfit for surgery [21]. A carefully performed ERCP with attention to the pancreatic and common bile duct anatomy up to the ampulla is critical. Histological confirmation is also essential since some normal papillas may appear to be polypoid. ERCP allows biopsies to be taken from the papilla and with cannulation, from the ampullary segment of the common bile duct or pancreatic duct. However, endoscopic biopsies cannot reliably exclude an invasive adenoma. False-negative results from endoscopic biopsies have been described in 25–60% of patients with carcinoma and diagnostic accuracy rates of 58–74% in reported series [2, 44–47]. Malignant foci are reported to occur in up to 15% or more of ampullary adenomas. Surgery has been advocated by some when endoscopic biopsies reveal high-grade dysplasia within an adenoma because of the risk of sampling error [46]. If the tumor arises from inside the ampulla of Vater it may not be completely visible at duodenoscopy. In such cases, an endoscopic sphinctero-tomy is necessary to expose the lesion and allow biopsies to be taken under direct visual control [48]. Because of the low accuracy rates of diagnostic endoscopic biopsies, some authors suggest obtaining a minimum number of six biopsies from the lesion in order to identify those patients in whom a surgical resection is more appropriate [20].

Endoscopic ultrasonography (EUS)

EUS is useful for tumor staging and assessing lymph node involvement and is advocated for large lesions and bulging intra-ampullary lesions [49]. EUS can accurately demonstrate extension of an ampullary lesion into the duodenal wall (T2) or into the pancreas (T3 or T4). Fine-needle aspiration biopsy (FNA) allows assessment of peri-lesional lymph nodes. EUS is not considered mandatory when planning endoscopic resection of small lesions [25,49–58].

Invasion of the muscularis mucosa and submucosal invasion can be determined with reasonable accuracy using intraductal ultrasound (IDUS). This technique involves the use of ultrasonic miniprobes inserted directly into the common bile duct or pancreatic duct [59].

EUS is a recommended technique for the staging of advanced neoplasms of the ampulla of Vater, especially prior to surgery. For early lesions, endoscopic snare resection followed by histological analysis of the resected specimen remains an accurate and effective method for evaluating curative endoscopic resection or the need for additional surgery.

Technique of endoscopic resection

Endoscopic snare resection of ampullary adenomas should be performed with the intent of completely excising all of the involved tissues. Although a relatively straightforward technique in expert hands, a number of different 'tricks' and variations in technique have been described to improve success rates of endoscopic resection and minimize complication rates. However, there is little if any prospective data on the efficacy of the various techniques that have been described in the literature.

Endoscopic retrograde cholangio-pancreatography (ERCP)

The endoscopic resection should be performed during ERCP. The addition of a few drops of methylene blue to the contrast agent used for cholangiography, helps to make it easier to identify the orifice of both the bile duct and pancreatic duct after snare excision. Theoretically, this may help to reduce the risk of post-ERCP pancreatitis by allowing quicker and safer cannulation of the bile and pancreatic duct, avoiding repeated cannulation and trauma to the main pancreatic duct.

Lifting of the lesion

Isolating the primary ampullary lesion by means of an injected submucosal fluid cushion (SFC) has been advocated by some endoscopists in order to reduce the risk of endoscopic perforation and bleeding after endoscopic papillectomy. If a 'non-lifting sign', or failure to lift the lesion away from the underlying submucosa, occurs, this may indicate an invasive lesion [23–25]. Endoscopic resection can be safely and even preferably performed without a SFC [20–22, 26,60]. The SFC will allow excision of the mucosal component of the ampullary adenoma leaving behind an intact sphincter of Oddi and underlying ampullary area with the attendant portions of the common bile duct and pancreatic duct. This can actually complicate the procedure by making subsequent cannulation of either the common bile duct or pancreatic duct technically very difficult. In case of lesions arising from within the ampulla of Vater, the SFC will interfere with en bloc resection [16,61]. An SFC may be useful for small lesions limited to and arising from a very flat papilla and when there is lateral (periampullary) spread of the lesion along the duodenal mucosa adjacent to the ampulla. Sometimes, the inferiorly spreading 'goatee' of neoplastic tissue on the lower part of the papilla and its frenulum can be resected safely by means of a pre-excision SFC. The inferior and laterally spreading components of the larger lesions are well suited to piecemeal snare-type EMR assisted by an SFC after the main or primary component of the ampullary lesion is removed by unassisted snare resection.

Resection of the ampullary lesion

Endoscopic resection is performed by snaring and removing the neoplasm and ampullary tissues down to the level of the muscularis propria [20]. Some endoscopists advocate performing a circumferential incision around the ampulla using a needle knife prior to endoscopic snare resection. This technique may facilitate accurate placement of the snare but entails risk and would require a SFC for added safety against perforation [23].

A variety of snares, including specially designed snares, may be used [17,62] (Fig. 8.5). In our unit a specially designed snare is used which is of monofilament construction, more flexible, and wider than standard snares to allow the snare to be accurately 'draped' around the lesion, preferably top down or from a proximal to distal approach. After the snare is tightened, the lesion is lifted up as it is excised under greater visual control. No more than 2 cm of tissue should be ensnared and excised in order to avoid a major complication such as

(b)

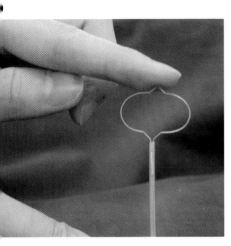
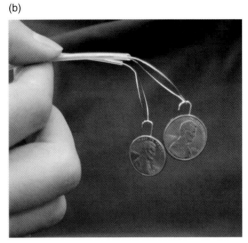

g. 8.5   (a) Specially designed ampullectomy snare which is monofilament and wider than a standard pol-
ectomy snare; (b) the snare is more flexible than a standard polypectomy snare, using a suspended penny
r weighted comparison. The flexibility allows the snare to be positioned accurately around the ampullary
ion.

perforation and bleeding. Larger lesions and especially those requiring palliation should be resected in a piecemeal fashion. There is no prospective data in
the literature comparing success rates for en bloc versus piecemeal resection of
ampullary tumors. In our experience the former method has most consistently
allowed complete resection. En bloc resection does allow for more accurate
histological evaluation of completeness of resection and depth of tumor invasion. Theoretically, en bloc resection may potentially reduce the risk of tumor
seeding post-resection although this remains to be determined. En bloc resection may also be associated with less thermal injury to the ampullary area, and
thus potentially a reduced risk of post-procedure pancreatitis [63,64]. In contrast, some experts advocate performing piecemeal resection in order to reduce
the risk of perforation and bleeding [24]. It is recommended that en bloc resection should always be performed when possible to reduce the risk of local
recurrence. When en bloc resection is not possible then residual adenomatous
tissue should be excised piecemeal during the same procedure [16,18,20–23,
27,28,60].

There is some debate as to the best method for snaring and grasping an
ampullary lesion. The majority of endoscopists advocate ensnaring the lesion
top down as mentioned above, from the proximal to the distal or caudal side
of the lesion. The apex of the snare is accurately placed at the superior margin
of the ampulla and the snare slowly closed while advancing the outer sheath of
the snare so as to impact and then grasp the entire base of the ampulla [25].
This maneuver is critical. There are no established recommendations as to the

power output or type of electro-surgical current. Some experts use a blended current whereas others recommend using a pure cutting current [16].

Additional thermal ablation

Any residual adenomatous tissue after attempted en bloc resection should be removed by either additional piecemeal snare resection or in some cases, additional thermal ablation may be necessary when snare resection is impossible, particularly for small fragments of residual tumor. Ablative thermal modalities include argon plasma coagulation, monopolar or multipolar electro-coagulation, and neodymium–yttrium aluminum garnet (Nd:YAG) laser. The preferred technique is largely dependent on equipment availability, local expertise, and personal preference of the endoscopist. Argon plasma coagulation has become a favored expeditious method for supplemental ablation of residual tissue. Thermal ablation should only be used as an adjunct to snare excision and not as a primary treatment. When thermal ablation is used for primary treatment of adenomas, specimens for histopathologic evaluation cannot be obtained and thus, the presence of cancer may be overlooked [16]. Primary thermal ablation can also result in obstruction of both the common bile duct and pancreatic ducts due to thermally induced edema and complications due to transient obstruction such as jaundice, cholangitis, and pancreatitis [8,26].

Pancreatic sphincterotomy and stenting

Acute pancreatitis is one of the most common and potentially severe, life-threatening complications. Pancreatitis is thought to occur as a result of edema and thermal injury to the pancreatic duct. Endoscopic pancreatic sphincterotomy and temporary pancreatic stent placement will maintain patency of the pancreatic duct and, thus, may reduce the risk of pancreatitis. There is some controversy over whether or not to stent the pancreatic duct after papillectomy. Some endoscopists advocate placing a pancreatic stent in all patients [23], whereas others advocate pancreatic stenting only [18,24,28,60] if there is delayed drainage of injected contrast [20,25,26]. Results from published trials have been inconclusive [17,26,65]. There has been only one published randomized study assessing the effects of pancreatic stenting on the incidence of pancreatitis after endoscopic papillectomy. This study was terminated early because of the high incidence of acute pancreatitis in patients who did not receive prophylactic pancreatic stenting (33%) [17]. The resultant small numbers of patients enrolled ($n = 19$) makes it difficult to draw definite conclusions [66].

Some authors prefer to use small, three or five French pancreatic stents without a proximal flap because of their tendency to migrate spontaneously

[17,22,24,26,67]. There has been some concern that larger diameter pancreatic stents may cause epithelial damage to the pancreatic duct [68–70]. However, the placement of a 3-Fr pancreatic stent can be difficult, requiring special expertise in handling very small guide-wires (0.018 in.), and until reasonable prospective data are available, larger stents (5–8.5-Fr diameter) are recommended [67]. Some endoscopists recommend leaving a pancreatic stent in place for at least one to two months before removal. Stenting, despite pancreatic sphincterotomy, will protect the pancreatic duct orifice during supplemental endoscopic resection or thermal ablation of any residual tumor [24]. The duration of stenting is unknown. The stents need only be left in place for several days to a week at most. In our experience at Mayo, stents are removed, if not spontaneously expelled, after one week. In patients who are available the day after the procedure, stent position is checked fluoroscopically and if still present, it is then extracted without sequelae [17].

Pancreatic sphincterotomy performed immediately after snare excision is recommended with or without pancreatic stenting. If there is immediate flow of pancreatic juice, instilled contrast promptly drains out, or air is seen within the pancreatic duct on fluoroscopy, then pancreatic stenting may be optional. Insertion of a naso-pancreatic drain for 24–48 h may be an alternative to pancreatic stenting. Pancreatic sphincterotomy, most importantly, may reduce the risk of subsequent, delayed fibrosis and stricturing of the pancreatic duct orifice [26].

Biliary sphincterotomy and stenting

In some cases, poor biliary drainage may be observed after papillectomy. In such cases, biliary drainage will be improved by performing biliary sphincterotomy either with or without subsequent biliary stenting. In general, biliary sphincterotomy is technically easier to perform than pancreatic sphincterotomy after resection. If there is incomplete drainage of bile and contrast after biliary sphincterotomy, then a large diameter biliary stent (10-Fr) should be placed and left for one to three months until repeat ERCP to identify any residual polyp and additional endoscopic therapy are planned [20]. There is little evidence for the role of endoscopic biliary sphincterotomy or stenting. Acute cholangitis rarely occurs immediately [16]. Biliary sphincterotomy may reduce the risk of infrequently occuring fibrosis and stenosis of the biliary orifice, which has been reported to occur in up to 10% of patients [16]. Both biliary and pancreatic sphincterotomy will open the ampullary bed and facilitate future surveillance of this area, especially in patients with FAP, who may require supplemental treatment which can easily be performed with minimal risk for complications.

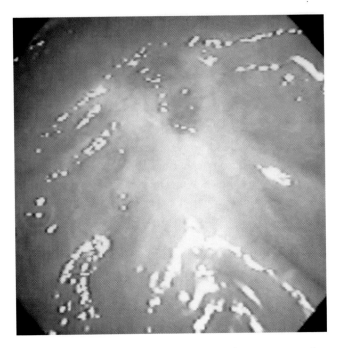

Fig. 8.6 An ampullary excision site in a patient with FAP without recurrent polyp at three years follow-up.

Outcomes

The success rate for endoscopic resection ranges between 74% and 92% (Fig. 8.6). The recurrence rate is reported to be between 0% and 33% [18–28,60]. The majority of published series involve small numbers of patients. Furthermore, it is difficult to compare and analyze the results of published series because of the retrospective nature of the studies with differences in the patient populations studied, indications for endoscopic papillectomy, differences in endoscopic technique, and histological data. Even the definition of 'success' varies from one study to another. Some authors consider the technical success of endoscopic resection whereas others report on the absence of local recurrence at long-term follow-up after resection. In addition, difficulty arises as to the definition of 'local recurrence' or 'residual adenoma' where there is biopsy-proven adenomatous tissue at endoscopic follow-up [16]. The majority of local recurrences are visible during the endoscopic follow-up, and can be easily treated endoscopically by additional snare excision or thermal treatment. Endoscopic treatment is minimally invasive and can be repeated indefinitely.

Adenomatous recurrence is more common in patients with FAP who are significantly younger and with smaller lesions compared to patients affected by sporadic tumors [22]. Other factors which may predict success rate at endoscopic papillectomy include masculine gender, age greater than 48 years, and lesions smaller than 24 mm in diameter [22].

Complications

The majority of complications following endoscopic papillectomy occur immediately. These are usually mild, requiring only medical or endoscopic treatment. The most common immediate complications are bleeding from the site of the papillectomy and acute pancreatitis; more rarely acute cholangitis and perforation may occur [16]. Mild self-limited bleeding is not uncommon immediately after resection. This might receive supplemental endoscopic therapy and should not be considered as a complication. The reported complication rate following endoscopic papillectomy varies between 10% and 58% (average rate 23%) [16–28,43,60]. The most common adverse event is bleeding, which may occur in up to 10% of procedures. Usually it is similar to the bleeding after endoscopic sphincterotomy, and may be managed by endoscopic measures such as the use of endoscopic hemostatic clips, epinephrine injection, or thermal coagulation. Acute pancreatitis occurs in up to 9% of patients, but in most cases is usually mild and treated conservatively. Retroperitoneal perforation is a rare complication of endoscopic papillectomy and is reported to occur in less than 1% of cases [16]. Too large a resection, or repeated free-hand attempts at pancreatic duct cannulation may increase the risk of retroperitoneal perforation. In most cases, these can be treated conservatively except where there are signs of sepsis, which requires surgical drainage via a posterior laparostomy [71].

Delayed complications are rare and are usually due to subsequent fibrosis and scarring at the site of the papillectomy causing stenosis of either the biliary and/or pancreatic duct orifice. In such cases, endoscopic therapy, with balloon dilatation of the duct orifice, is usually successful. Mortality following endoscopic papillectomy is rare with a reported incidence of up to 0.4% [16].

Surveillance after ESP

Currently, there are no recommended guidelines on the optimal time interval for surveillance following endoscopic resection. However, all patients should be followed up regularly to determine whether or not resection is complete, and to identify and treat any areas of local recurrence. The timing between endoscopic resection and the first follow-up examination to some extent depends on the personal preferences of the endoscopist performing the resection, the success rate of complete excision, and histological analysis of the excised specimen. In patients where a piecemeal resection has been performed, when the resection margins of the lesion are involved by tumor, or in cases of adenoma with high-grade dysplasia or invasive carcinoma, repeat examination should be performed early at one to three months post-resection. In contrast, in patients with adenoma with low-grade dysplasia and en bloc complete excision with histological evidence of tumor-free margins, follow-up examination may be delayed six to twelve months post-resection [22].

Endoscopic resection is considered complete when there is no visible residual adenoma or recurrence after a follow-up examination with biopsy. In cases of incomplete tumor excision, repeated endoscopic excision (with snare or biopsies forceps) or thermal ablation (argon plasma coagulation) should be performed at 2–3 month intervals until any residual tumor tissue has been completely ablated [22]. In contrast, for lesions which are completely excised following initial resection, surveillance endoscopy and multiple biopsies should be performed at six to twelve monthly intervals for a minimum of two years [22]. In patients with sporadic adenomas, the risk of local recurrence after two years is extremely low and in such cases some authors would advocate only repeating endoscopic examinations if clinically indicated [20]. Others, however, would recommend continued regular surveillance at yearly intervals [20,21,23,28,60,64]. In our experience at Mayo, patients with sporadic adenomas will have surveillance continued for five years. In contrast, in patients with FAP who have no evidence of local recurrence, the ampullary region should undergo periodic lifelong endoscopic surveillance at established intervals, along with biopsy, which can be as long as three years in the presence of complete eradication that has been histologically proven [22].

Video legend

Two video segments are presented with similar-sized lesions in a patient with FAP and a sporadic adenoma. The lesions are 1–1.5 cm in size. In the first video there is a classic 'goatee' extension of the adenoma inferiorly below the adenomatous area and enlarged papilla of Vater. The ERCP cholangiogram is shown prior to snare resection. This demonstrates an uninvolved distal common bile duct. Snare excision is performed using a specialized ampullectomy snare positioned in a 'top down' fashion. After the main component of the adenoma is excised, a biliary sphincterotomy is performed followed by placement of a 5-French single pigtail pancreatic stent for prophylaxis from pancreatitis. Supplemental cautery is performed using an 0.035 inch fistulatome. In the second video, the accurate placement of the snare is emphasized, lifting the ensnared lesion upward to examine the positioning of the monofilament snare wire. Post-excision ERCP and biliary sphincterotomy is also demonstrated through an intact residual biliary component of the sphincter of Oddi.

References

1 Scarpa A, Capelli P, Zamboni G *et al.* Neoplasia of the ampulla of Vater. Ki-ras and p53 mutations. *Am J Pathol* 1993; **142**: 1163–72.

2 Beger HG, Treitschke F, Gansauge F, Harada N, Hiki N, Mattfeldt T. Tumor of the ampulla of Vater: experience with local or radical resection in 171 consecutively treated patients. *Arch Surg* 1999; **134**: 526–32.

3 Park SW, Song SY, Chung JB, Lee SK, Moon YM, Kang JK, Park IS. Endoscopic snare resection for tumors of the ampulla of Vater. *Yonsei Med J* 2000; **41**: 213–18.

4 Stolte M, Pscherer C. Adenoma-carcinoma sequence in the papilla of Vater. *Scand J Gastroenterol* 1996; **31**: 376–82.

5 Kaiser A, Jurowich C, Schonekas H, Gebhardt C, Wunsch PH. The adenoma-carcinoma sequence applies to epithelial tumours of the papilla of Vater. *Z Gastroenterol* 2002; **40**: 913–20.

6 Burke CA, Beck GJ, Church JM, van Stolk RU. The natural history of untreated duodenal and ampullary adenomas in patients with familial adenomatous polyposis followed in an endoscopic surveillance program. *Gastrointest Endosc* 1999; **49**: 358–64.

7 Ouaissi M, Panis Y, Sielezneff I *et al.* Long-term outcome after ampullectomy for ampullary lesions associated with familial adenomatous polyposis. *Dis Colon Rectum* 2005; **48**: 2192–6.

8 Bleau BL, Gostout CJ. Endoscopic treatment of ampullary adenomas in familial adenomatous polyposis. *J Clin Gastroenterol* 1996; **22(3)**: 237–41.

9 Klempnauer J, Ridder GJ, Maschek H, Pichlmayr R. Carcinoma of the ampulla of Vater: determinants of long-term survival in 94 resected patients. *HPB Surg* 1998; **11**: 1–11.

10 Branum GD, Pappas TN, Meyers WC. The management of tumors of the ampulla of Vater by local resection. *Ann Surg* 1996; **224**: 621–7.

11 Brown KM, Tompkins AJ, Yong S, Aranha GV, Shoup M. Pancreaticoduodenectomy is curative in the majority of patients with node-negative ampullary cancer. *Arch Surg* 2005; **140**: 529–32.

12 Todoroki T, Koike N, Morishita Y, Kawamoto T, Ohkohchi N, Shoda J, Fukuda Y, Takahashi H. Patterns and predictors of failure after curative resections of carcinoma of the ampulla of Vater. *Ann Surg Oncol* 2003; **10**: 1176–83.

13 Di Giorgio A, Alfieri S, Rotondi F *et al.* Pancreatoduodenectomy for tumors of Vater's ampulla: report on 94 consecutive patients. *World J Surg* 2005; **29**: 513–18.

14 Schmidt CM, Powell ES, Yiannoutsos CT *et al.* Pancreaticoduodenectomy: a 20-year experience in 516 patients. *Arch Surg* 2004; **139**: 718–25.

15 Yeo CJ, Cameron JL, Sohn TA *et al.* Six hundred fifty consecutive pancreaticoduodenectomies in the 1990s: pathology, complications, and outcomes. *Ann Surg* 1997; **226**: 248–57.

16 Han J, Kim MH. Endoscopic papillectomy for adenomas of the major duodenal papilla (with video). *Gastrointest Endosc* 2006; **63**: 292–301.

17 Harewood GC, Pochron NL, Gostout CJ. Prospective, randomized, controlled trial of prophylactic pancreatic stent placement for endoscopic snare excision of the duodenal ampulla. *Gastrointest Endosc* 2005; **62**: 367–70.

18 Maguchi H, Takahashi K, Katanuma A, Hayashi T, Yoshida A. Indication of endoscopic papillectomy for tumors of the papilla of Vater and its problems. *Dig Endosc* 2003; **15**: S33.

19 Bertoni G, Sassatelli R, Nigrisoli E, Bedogni G. Endoscopic snare papillectomy in patients with familial adenomatous polyposis and ampullary adenoma. *Endoscopy* 1997; **29**: 685–8.

20 Binmoeller KF, Boaventura S, Ramsperger K, Soehendra N. Endoscopic snare excision of benign adenomas of the papilla of Vater. *Gastrointest Endosc* 1993; **39**: 127–31.

21 Bohnacker S, Seitz U, Nguyen D *et al.* Endoscopic resection of benign tumors of the duodenal papilla without and with intraductal growth. *Gastrointest Endosc* 2005; **62**: 551–60.

22 Catalano MF, Linder JD, Chak A *et al.* Endoscopic management of adenoma of the major duodenal papilla. *Gastrointest Endosc* 2004; **59**: 225–32.

23 Cheng CL, Sherman S, Fogel EL *et al.* Endoscopic snare papillectomy for tumors of the duodenal papillae. *Gastrointest Endosc* 2004; **60**: 757–64.

24 Desilets DJ, Dy RM, Ku PM *et al.* Endoscopic management of tumors of the major duodenal papilla: refined techniques to improve outcome and avoid complications. *Gastrointest Endosc* 2001; **54**: 202–08.

25 Kahaleh M, Shami VM, Brock A *et al*. Factors predictive of malignancy and endoscopic resectability in ampullary neoplasia. *Am J Gastroenterol* 2004; **99**: 2335–9.

26 Norton ID, Gostout CJ, Baron TH, Geller A, Petersen BT, Wiersema MJ. Safety and outcome of endoscopic snare excision of the major duodenal papilla. *Gastrointest Endosc* 2002; **56**: 239–43.

27 Saurin JC, Chavaillon A, Napoleon B *et al*. Long-term follow-up of patients with endoscopic treatment of sporadic adenomas of the papilla of Vater. *Endoscopy* 2003; **35**: 402–6.

28 Zadorova Z, Dvofak M, Hajer J. Endoscopic therapy of benign tumors of the papilla of Vater. *Endoscopy* 2001; **33**: 345–7.

29 Bohnacker S, Soehendra N, Maguchi H, Chung JB, Howell DA. Endoscopic resection of benign tumors of the papilla of Vater. *Endoscopy* 2006; **4**: 521–5.

30 Yoon YS, Kim SW, Park SJ *et al*. Clinicopathologic analysis of early ampullary cancers with a focus on the feasibility of ampullectomy. *Ann Surg* 2005; **242**: 92–100.

31 Yoshida T, Matsumoto T, Shibata K *et al*. Patterns of lymph node metastasis in carcinoma of the ampulla of Vater. *Hepatogastroenterology* 2000; **47**: 880–3.

32 Guindi M, Riddell RH. The pathology of epithelial pre-malignancy of the gastrointestinal tract. *Best Pract Res Clin Gastroenterol* 2001; **15**: 191–210.

33 Komorowski RA, Beggs BK, Geenan JE, Venu RP. Assessment of ampulla of Vater pathology. An endoscopic approach. *Am J Surg Pathol* 1991; **15**: 1188–96.

34 Schlemper RJ, Riddell RH, Kato Y *et al*. The Vienna classification of gastrointestinal epithelial neoplasia. *Gut* 2000; **47**: 251–5.

35 Stolte M. The new Vienna classification of epithelial neoplasia of the gastrointestinal tract: advantages and disadvantages. *Virchows Arch* 2003; **442**: 99–106.

36 Rattner DW, Fernandez-del Castillo C, Brugge WR, Warshaw AL. Defining the criteria for local resection of ampullary neoplasms. *Arch Surg* 1996; **131**: 366–71.

37 Sawada T, Muto T. Familial adenomatous polyposis: should patients undergo surveillance of the upper gastrointestinal tract? *Endoscopy* 1995; **27**: 6–11.

38 Matsumoto T, Iida M, Nakamura S *et al*. Natural history of ampullary adenoma in familial adenomatous polyposis: reconfirmation of benign nature during extended surveillance. *Am J Gastroenterol* 2000; **95**: 1557–62.

39 Iida M, Yao T, Itoh H *et al*. Natural history of duodenal lesions in Japanese patients with familial adenomatosis coli (Gardner's syndrome). *Gastroenterology* 1989; **96**: 1301–6.

40 Noda Y, Watanabe H, Iida M *et al*. Histologic follow-up of ampullary adenomas in patients with familial adenomatosis coli. *Cancer* 1992; **70**: 1847–56.

41 Burke CA, Beck GJ, Church JM, van Stolk RU. The natural history of untreated duodenal and ampullary adenomas in patients with familial adenomatous polyposis followed in an endoscopic surveillance program. *Gastrointest Endosc* 1999; **49**: 358–64.

42 Shemesh E, Bat L. A prospective evaluation of the upper gastrointestinal tract and periampullary region in patients with Gardner syndrome. *Am J Gastroenterol* 1985; **80**: 825–7.

43 Martin JA, Haber GB. Ampullary adenoma: clinical manifestations, diagnosis, and treatment. *Gastrointest Endosc Clin N Am* 2003; **13**: 649–69.

44 Sauvanet A, Chapuis O, Hammel P *et al*. Are endoscopic procedures able to predict the benignity of ampullary tumors? *Am J Surg* 1997; **174**: 355–8.

45 Yamaguchi K, Enjoji M, Kitamura K. Endoscopic biopsy has limited accuracy in diagnosis of ampullary tumors. *Gastrointest Endosc* 1990; **36**: 588–92.

46 Meneghetti AT, Safadi B, Stewart L, Way LW. Local resection of ampullary tumors. *J Gastrointest Surg* 2005; **9**: 1300–6.

47 de Castro SM, van Heek T, Kuhlmann KF *et al*. Surgical management of neoplasms of the ampulla of Vater: local resection or pancreatoduodenectomy and prognostic factors for survival. *Surgery* 2004; **136**: 994–1002.

48 Bourgeois N, Dunham F, Verhest A, Cremer M. Endoscopic biopsies of the papilla of Vater at the time of endoscopic sphincterotomy: difficulties in interpretation. *Gastrointest Endosc* 1984; **30**: 163–6.

49 Yasuda K, Mukai H, Cho E, Nakajima M, Kawai K. The use of endoscopic ultrasonography in the diagnosis and staging of carcinoma of the papilla of Vater. *Endoscopy* 1988; **20 Suppl 1**: 218–22.

50 Buscail L, Pages P, Berthelemy P, Fourtanier G, Frexinos J, Escourrou J. Role of EUS in the management of pancreatic and ampullary carcinoma: a prospective study assessing resectability and prognosis. *Gastrointest Endosc* 1999; **50**: 34–40.

51 Cannon ME, Carpenter SL, Elta GH *et al*. EUS compared with CT, magnetic resonance imaging, and angiography and the influence of biliary stenting on staging accuracy of ampullary neoplasms. *Gastrointest Endosc* 1999; **50**: 27–33.

52 Chen CH, Tseng LJ, Yang CC, Yeh YH, Mo LR. The accuracy of endoscopic ultrasound, endoscopic retrograde cholangiopancreatography, computed tomography, and transabdominal ultrasound in the detection and staging of primary ampullary tumors. *Hepatogastroenterology* 2001; **48**: 1750–3.

53 Kubo H, Chijiiwa Y, Akahoshi K, Hamada S, Matsui N, Nawata H. Pre-operative staging of ampullary tumours by endoscopic ultrasound. *Br J Radiol* 1999; **72**: 443–7.

54 Maluf-Filho F, Sakai P, Cunha JE *et al*. Radial endoscopic ultrasound and spiral computed tomography in the diagnosis and staging of periampullary tumors. *Pancreatology* 2004; **4**: 122–8.

55 Menzel J, Hoepffner N, Sulkowski U *et al*. Polypoid tumors of the major duodenal papilla: preoperative staging with intraductal US, EUS, and CT – a prospective, histopathologically controlled study. *Gastrointest Endosc* 1999; **49**: 349–57.

56 Midwinter MJ, Beveridge CJ, Wilsdon JB, Bennett MK, Baudouin CJ, Charnley RM. Correlation between spiral computed tomography, endoscopic ultrasonography and findings at operation in pancreatic and ampullary tumours. *Br J Surg* 1999; **86**: 189–93.

57 Skordilis P, Mouzas IA, Dimoulios PD, Alexandrakis G, Moschandrea J, Kouroumalis E. Is endosonography an effective method for detection and local staging of the ampullary carcinoma? A prospective study. *BMC Surg* 2002; **2**: 1.

58 Tio TL, Sie LH, Kallimanis G *et al*. Staging of ampullary and pancreatic carcinoma: comparison between endosonography and surgery. *Gastrointest Endosc* 1996; **44**: 706–13.

59 Itoh A, Goto H, Naitoh Y, Hirooka Y, Furukawa T, Hayakawa T. Intraductal ultrasonography in diagnosing tumor extension of cancer of the papilla of Vater. *Gastrointest Endosc* 1997; **45**: 251–60.

60 Vogt M, Jakobs R, Benz C, Arnold JC, Adamek HE, Riemann JF. Endoscopic therapy of adenomas of the papilla of Vater. A retrospective analysis with long-term follow-up. *Dig Liver Dis* 2000; **32**: 339–45.

61 Wong RF, DiSario JA. Approaches to endoscopic ampullectomy. *Curr Opin Gastroenterol* 2004; **20**: 460–7.

62 Soehendra N, Binmoeller KF, Bohnacker S *et al*. Endoscopic snare mucosectomy in the esophagus without any additional equipment: a simple technique for resection of flat early cancer. *Endoscopy* 1997; **29**: 380–3.

63 Aiura K, Imaeda H, Kitajima M, Kumai K. Balloon-catheter-assisted endoscopic snare papillectomy for benign tumors of the major duodenal papilla. *Gastrointest Endosc* 2003; **57**: 743–7.

64 Charton JP, Deinert K, Schumacher B, Neuhaus H. Endoscopic resection for neoplastic diseases of the papilla of Vater. *J Hepatobiliary Pancreat Surg* 2004; **11**: 245–51.

65 Fujita N, Noda Y, Kobayashi G, Kimura K, Ito K. Endoscopic papillectomy: is there room for this procedure in clinical practice? *Dig Endosc* 2003; **15**: 253–5.

66 Baillie J. Endoscopic ampullectomy: does pancreatic stent placement make it safer? *Gastrointest Endosc* 2005; **62**: 371–3.

67 Baillie J. Endoscopic ampullectomy. *Am J Gastroenterol* 2005; **100**: 2379–81.

68 Rashdan A, Fogel EL, McHenry L, Jr., Sherman S, Temkit M, Lehman GA. Improved stent characteristics for prophylaxis of post-ERCP pancreatitis. *Clin Gastroenterol Hepatol* 2004; **2**: 322–9.

69 Sherman S, Alvarez C, Robert M, Ashley SW, Reber HA, Lehman GA. Polyethylene pancreatic duct stent-induced changes in the normal dog pancreas. *Gastrointest Endosc* 1993; **39**: 658–64.

70 Smith MT, Sherman S, Ikenberry SO, Hawes RH, Lehman GA. Alterations in pancreatic ductal morphology following polyethylene pancreatic stent therapy. *Gastrointest Endosc* 1996; **44**: 268–75.

71 Doglietto GB, Pacelli F, Caprino P, Alfieri S, Tortorelli AP, Mutignani M. Posterior laparostomy through the bed of the 12th rib to drain retroperitoneal infection after endoscopic sphincterotomy. *Br J Surg* 2004; **91**: 730–3.

CHAPTER 9

EMR for Colorectal Lesions

ALESSANDRO REPICI, GIUSEPPE DE CARO,
CARMELO LUIGIANO, AND RICCARDO ROSATI

Introduction

The removal of colon polyps is the commonest therapeutic maneuver in the large bowel. The technique for small or large polyps is basically the same with repetitive but similar action required for larger polyps. Open access endoscopy and screening programs have been recently introduced in Western countries and have led to the detection of an increased number of lesions in the early stages of neoplastic transformation. Unfortunately polyps larger than 3 cm, involving more than one-third of circumference or two haustral folds or with a flat/depressed morphology are more challenging to remove with the standard polypectomy technique and usually require a different endoscopic approach, which has been named endoscopic mucosal resection (EMR). EMR is now an established technique that tremendously extends the ability to remove in a minimally invasive way colonic lesions that would otherwise require surgical or ablative therapies. One more important advantage of EMR over standard polypectomy is that EMR has the potential to provide en bloc resection specimens for histopathologic analysis. The plane of resection during EMR is typically the middle-to-deep submucosal layer as compared with standard polypectomy which normally provides a resection at a mucosal level.

This chapter will review current data regarding the technique and patient selection as well as complications and outcomes of endoscopic mucosal resection for colonic lesions.

Endoscopic Mucosal Resection. Edited by M. Conio, P. Siersema, A. Repici and T. Ponchon. © 2008 Blackwell Publishing. ISBN 978-1-4051-5885-5.

Concepts of early colorectal cancer

Early colorectal cancer is defined by the Japanese rule as being limited to the mucosa or invading only to the submucosa, regardless of the presence or absence of lymph node metastases [1].

From an endoscopic point of view, in the colon, neoplastic lesions are called 'superficial' at endoscopy when the endoscopic appearance suggests either a small cancer or a non-invasive neoplastic lesion (dysplasia/adenoma). If invasive, 'superficial' tumors correspond to the T1 stage of the TNM classification, in which invasion is limited to the mucosa and submucosa. 'Superficial' tumors are typically non-obstructive, usually are asymptomatic, and often are detected as an incidental finding or by screening [2].

The macroscopic classification system provided by the Japanese Research Society for Cancer of the Colon and Rectum (JRSC) divides the gross appearances of early colorectal neoplasms into three categories: protruded or polypoid, flat elevated, and depressed [3]. The Paris classification [4] is an extension of the previously used Japanese Classification of Colorectal Carcinoma. These classifications serve as useful guides to distinguish lesions amenable to endoscopic therapy.

The polypoid type consists of the pedunculated or semipedunculated (type 0–Ip) and sessile (0–Is) morphology. The non-polypoid type comprises slightly elevated (0–IIa), completely flat (0–IIb), and slightly depressed (without ulcer) (0–IIc) lesions. Excavated or ulcerated superficial lesions (type 0-III) are practically non-existent in the colon, and this type of lesion is described primarily in gastric cancer.

However, these classifications are still poorly standardized, leading to significant differences in the interpretation and definition of non-polypoid colonic lesions with problems in interobserver agreement and substantial differences between Western and Japanese experiences [5] and even from endoscopists of the same area.

The original description of a flat neoplasm by Muto et al. [6] in 1985 is of a lesion slightly elevated above the mucosa with a reddish surface and/or a central depression that is seen after the lumen has been adequately inflated. An alternative definition describes these lesions as mucosal elevations with a flat or partially rounded surface where the height is less than half its diameter [7] or histologically as those in which the thickness of the lesion is less than twice that of the adjacent normal colonic mucosa [8]. The depressed-type colon cancer was first described in 1977 [9,10] by Japanese authors. The occurrence of this lesion is now widely accepted and is reported throughout the world with an increasing incidence even in Western countries.

Recognition of depression is very important because depressed lesions are often associated with invasive cancer even when they are very small. The depressed-type colorectal cancers either can be absolutely depressed or accompanied by a slightly elevated margin [9]. Some lesions with depression are elevated as a result of submucosal invasion and proliferation of the tumor cells [10]. Such lesions must not be mistaken for ordinary elevated neoplasms because they are quite different from each other in biological behavior.

Chromoscopy is useful for confirming flat and depressed colorectal lesions, for determining their lateral extent, and for clarifying their gross configuration; this is useful especially in determining the presence or absence of depression within the lesions.

There is some confusion about the depressed and flat lesions. Lesions that are called *flat* adenomas are not absolutely flat, but often are elevated slightly. It is true that some adenomas appear to have a depression and resemble depressed-type early cancers; the depression in a true depressed lesion is rather extensive and clearly demarcated. In contrast, the depression in flat elevated adenomas actually is an ill-defined pseudodepression with only a thorny or groove-like appearance [11]. Depressed lesions are not part of flat adenomas but should be regarded as a different entity, because the latter almost invariably are benign. Invasive rates in flat elevated adenomas are slightly lower than but not remarkably different from those in protruded polyps [7]. Flat lesions are usually benign or only focally malignant and grow very slowly, not becoming invasive until they are rather large. In contrast, depressed lesions apparently grow rather rapidly, advancing at an early stage [12] and most of the time are not suitable for endoscopic resection. The depressed-type lesions are reported not to have K-*ras* point mutation, although their genetic alterations are not clear [13] and it is certain that they arise without adenoma-carcinoma sequence [14].

In addition to the Japanese macroscopic classification of early neoplastic lesion, flat adenomas are further classified according to their size. Laterally spreading tumors are defined as those flat adenomas larger than 10 mm in diameter which extend circumferentially rather than vertically [15]. This category is further divided into a granular type, which is composed of fine granules, and a non-granular type (Fig. 9.1(a),(b)), which is devoid of apparent nodules or granules and seems to have higher incidence of cancer with submucosal invasion [16].

The role of EMR in the treatment of early cancer of the colon is becoming more and more well defined, following the guidelines of the Japanese Society of Digestive Endoscopy inclusion criteria, which are: adenoma and small well-differentiated carcinoma; confined to the mucosa or cancer with minimal invasion to submucosa; and without any invasion to lymphatic channels or vessels [17].

(a)

(b)

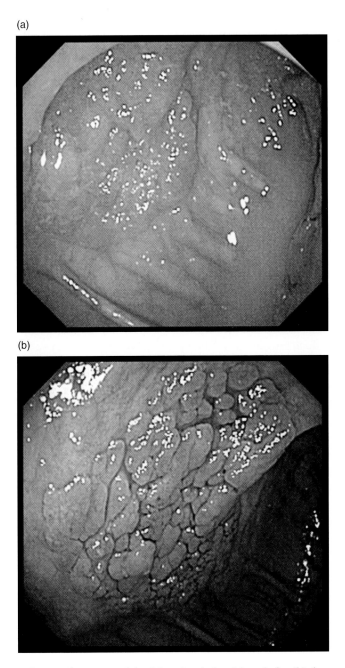

Fig. 9.1 Laterally spreading tumor of the right colon, before (a), and after (b) chromoscopy with indigocarmine.

Endoscopic diagnosis and staging of early colorectal cancers

Early colorectal cancers are usually without symptoms and their identification depends on the knowledge of their endoscopic morphology. In many cases high-grade dysplasia and adenocarcinoma are not identifiable during an endoscopic session, and for this reason the endoscopists should use additional technology to increase the sensitivity of the endoscopic investigation.

The evolution in the last years of technology applied to endoscopy have increased the possibility of detection and characterization of lesions of gastrointestinal mucosa.

The ability to magnify endoscopic images in real time by using magnification endoscopy permits the identification of microscopic lesions of the mucosa that cannot be seen with standard endoscopy.

A role of a combination of chromoendoscopy with indigocarmine and magnification endoscopy in the colon has been suggested for the diagnosis of flat and depressed lesions, identification of dysplasia, discrimination among polyp types, and assessing completeness of EMR.

With magnification, the openings of colonic crypts are referred to as pits, and the specific arrangement of the openings of the glands in various kinds of lesions is called the 'pit pattern', which shows strong correlation with the histopathological appearance [18].

Kudo has also proposed a classification of the fine surface structure of the mucosa, as well as that of small lesions, into pit pattern types I to V after vital staining especially with indigo carmine [19,20]. One of the most important challenges of endoscopic pit pattern diagnosis remains the differential diagnosis between non-neoplastic and neoplastic lesions.

Lesions with type I and II pit patterns obviate any necessity for endoscopic resection because of their negativity for neoplasia. Lesions with type IIIs (small), IIIl (large), or IV pit patterns could be treated endoscopically because they are probably adenomatous but not invasive. Lesions with type Vn (non-structural) pit pattern should be treated surgically because they are invasive and may have nodal metastases. Lesions with type Vi (irregular) pit pattern include a number of lesions from benign adenoma to invasive carcinoma; these kind of lesions are first treated endoscopically, and additional surgical colectomy and lymph node dissection are considered after the histological analysis of the biopsy specimen; non-invasive or minimally invasive (sm 1a) lesions without vessels infiltration can be only observed [21]. The ability to distinguish neoplastic from non-neoplastic lesions has been reported with a sensitivity and a specificity of more than 90% [22].

The potential of EUS evaluation before colonic EMR remains controversial.

High-frequency-miniprobe ultrasound (HFUP) has the ability to distinguish the colorectal mucosa as a nine-layered structure and hence provide an in vivo staging tool. In a prospective study Harada *et al.* [23] determined the utility of endoscopic ultrasonography in colonic EMR by using a 15 MHz miniprobe to assess submucosal invasion in 35 patients who were considered for endoscopic therapy. EUS resulted in suboptimal measuring of the precise depth of submucosal involvement. It was able to clearly distinguish shallow from deep invasion and thus determine suitability for EMR (86% accuracy). Ninety-two per cent of cancers thought to be unresectable on EUS were unresectable, whereas only 70% of cancers that were thought to be superficial were in fact resectable. Thus, EUS has better predictive value for deep, unresectable lesions.

Similarly, Hizawa *et al.* concluded that EUS could not be relied upon to determine the appropriate treatment for early colorectal cancer [24]. The reported accuracy of the invasion depth diagnosis from the largest series by Saitoh *et al.* was around 80% [25].

Due to these conflicting results EUS is not currently used before EMR for colonic lesions in many centers.

A simple and cheap method to evaluate the submucosal infiltration of early colonic neoplasms is 'the non-lifting sign' that has been proposed by Uno *et al.* [26]. Fluid is injected beneath the lesion at endoscopy. For those lesions with invasion into the deeper layers of the submucosa, the desmoplastic response prevents injected fluid from infiltrating underneath the tumor, so that the neighboring normal mucosa elevates but the lesion itself does not, resulting in the 'non-lifting sign'. When the sign is negative, the lesion is elevated and suitable for immediate endoscopic mucosal resection (EMR).

Lesions that show the non-lifting sign are not suitable for EMR, and should be tattooed with India ink to aid identification at surgery as small flat cancers may not be palpable at laparotomy [27].

Placement of tattoos above and below the lesion are recommended to aid localization by both the surgeon and the histopathologist.

Narrow band imaging (NBI) is a high-resolution endoscopic procedure that enhances the structure of the mucosal surface without the injection of any substances.

NBI enables better visualization of the mucosal patterns because blue light allows for optimal superficial imaging; moreover NBI reveals the superficial vasculature because of absorption of the blue light by haemoglobin (Fig. 9.2(a),(b)).

Machida *et al.*, in a pilot study performed between November 2001 and August 2002, enlisted 34 patients (22 men and 12 women) who were being followed up in an endoscopic surveillance program [28]. The detected lesions were each investigated three times, first by conventional colonoscopy, next by NBI colonoscopy and lastly, by chromoendoscopy using 0.2% indigo carmine dye. A total of 43 colorectal lesions were evaluated in the 34 patients. Compared with conventional colonoscopy, the pit pattern observed during

(a)

(b)

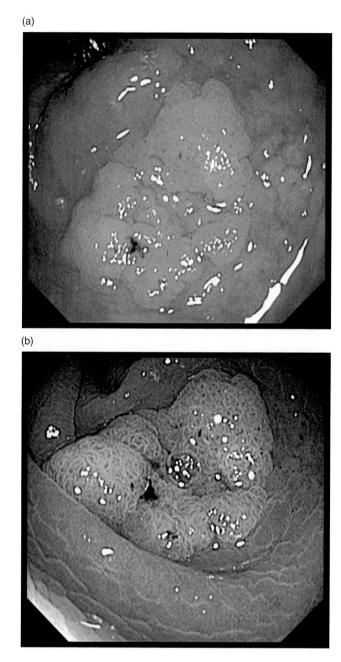

Fig. 9.2 Flat adenoma of the left colon (a), same image after NBI (b).

magnifying colonoscopy was better visualized by NBI ($p < 0.001$). The accuracy of endoscopic diagnosis compared with the histological findings was 79.1% for conventional endoscopy, in contrast to NBI colonoscopy (93.4%). NBI colonoscopy had a sensitivity of 100% and a specificity of 75% in the differentiation of neoplastic and non-neoplastic lesion [28].

Optical coherence tomography (OCT) is an emerging medical imaging technology that relies on the backscattering of light to obtain cross-sectional images of tissue.

This method is similar to ultrasonography but it uses light waves rather than acoustical waves. OCT permits the visualization in real time of the mucosa, the muscularis mucosae, and the superficial layer of submucosa.

Cho *et al.* [29] found that due to interference, the probe provided little benefit in imaging neoplastic lesions, but interesting views of the superficial colonic wall were obtained in patients with teleangectasia and ischemic colitis.

Confocal laser endoscopy is a technique that uses a confocal laser with a wavelength of 488 nanometers. With this method it is possible to visualize single cells and glands of the superficial epithelium, using fluorescein sodium as a contrast agent.

Fluorescein was used for the prospective component of the initial study, in which 42 patients with indications for screening or surveillance colonoscopy after previous polypectomy underwent colonoscopy. A total of 13 020 confocal images from 390 different locations were compared with the histological data from 1038 biopsies. With the newly developed confocal pattern classification, it was possible to predict the presence of neoplastic changes with a high degree of accuracy: sensitivity 97.4%, specificity 99.4%, accuracy 99.2% [30].

Techniques of EMR for early colorectal lesions

Endoscopic mucosal resection is a major advancement in endoscopy. In contrast to what is currently believed by the majority of endoscopists, mucosectomy was not invented in Japan. It was originally described by Deyle *et al.* [31] as early as 1973, and has been sophisticated and widely used by many others, especially Japanese endoscopists, since then.

The achievement of a proper position in front of the polyp is a crucial issue to success with the EMR of colonic lesions. It is often considerably easier to pass the scope far beyond the polyp, even to the cecum and attempt EMR during the withdrawal phase of the examination; as the scope is withdrawn, the loops are removed and the polyp, which proved difficult to position during intubation, may be quite easily approached. Once the colonoscope has been straightened, the ability to torque the instrument and freely use dial controls is restored, permitting the examiner to precisely maneuver the devices around the target lesions.

An alternative technique for removal of lesions located on the far side of a fold is to perform a U-turn maneuver. This can be accomplished in the cecum, proximal ascending colon, and occasionally in the transverse colon. It is more difficult to resect a polyp in a U-turn mode because the tip deflection responses are opposite to those usually expected. In such a case a narrow caliber endoscope such as a therapeutic gastroscope or a variable stiffness pediatric scope may permit easier polypectomy. The major attribute of these small caliber scopes is that they have a tighter bending radius of the tip than does a standard colonoscope.

Submucosal injection is a major step in performing colorectal EMR. A variety of solutions have been used to create a submucosal cushion including normal (physiologic) saline (NSS), hypertonic saline (3%), hypertonic glucose (D50), glycerol solutions, and diluted epinephrine solution (1:10000). Most practitioners use NSS. Interest in other agents is in an effort to prolong the 'pillow-effect' and decrease the risk of bleeding, transmural burn syndrome, and perforation (Fig. 9.3(a)–(e)).

There are still insufficient data to identify the ideal solution even on the base of a cost-effectiveness evaluation.

If a more viscous solution such as hyaluronic acid must be injected it may be very helpful to use a large channel needle 21 or 20 gauge. The needle should be directed adjacent to the base of the lesion at a 45° to the bowel wall in order to correctly penetrate just below the lesion and inject the solution into the submucosal layer beneath the lesion. If no cushion is observed, the needle may be too superficial or too deep and needs to be adjusted accordingly. Only the submucosal layer will expand with fluid injection.

When injecting around the circumference of a lesion, or for lesions draped over a fold, it is advantageous to inject at the far aspect of the lesion first to maintain or enhance its visualization. Injecting directly through the lesion should be avoided when possible because it carries the theoretical risk of contributing to metastasis even though up to now there has been no reported case of malignant cells spreading due to submucosal injection.

Whatever is the selected technique of EMR, either a blended current or pure coagulation current could be used. Unfortunately no previous studies have reported comparative data to support one or the other mode when performing EMR. A comparison of blended versus continuous coagulation current for pedunculated colorectal polyps failed to show a statistically significant difference in the incidence of major complications such as bleeding, transmural burn, and perforation [32]. The timing of major bleeding, however, was significantly different: all of the major hemorrhages were immediate when blended current was used; all were delayed (2–8 days) when pure coagulation current was used. Our group and some others suggest that a combination of blended and coagulation current may be safely used for colonic EMR because the

(a)

(b)

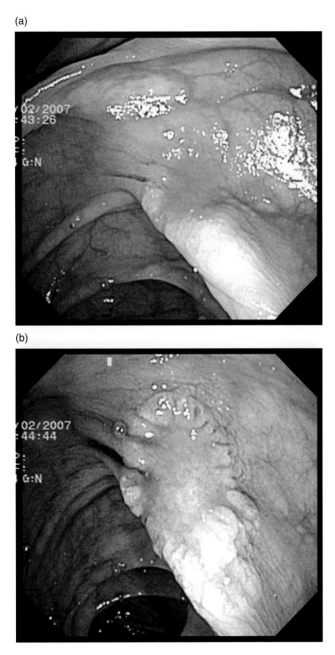

Fig. 9.3 A small flat adenoma with central depression (a), after chromoendoscopy (b), lifted with saline (c) and resected (d and e).

(c)

(d)

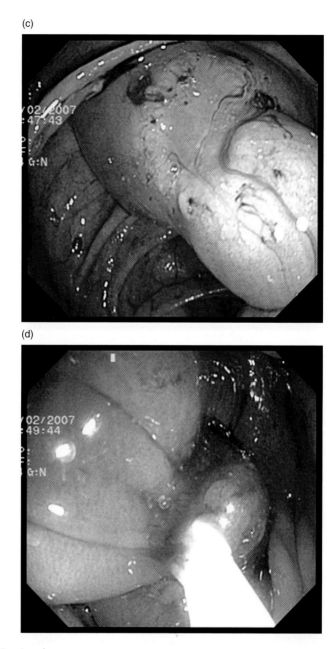

Fig. 9.3 Continued

introduction of a saline pillow protects against transmural injury, whereas the risk of acute and delayed bleeding is diminished [33–35].

Once the lesion has been raised, a snare is applied over the lesion and closed. Applying suction as the snare is closed helps in retaining the mucosa within the snare. Once the lesion is caught in the snare, the snare is relaxed slightly to

(e)

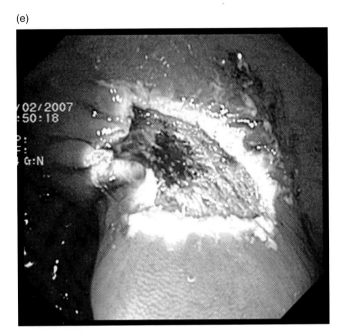

Fig. 9.3   Continued

allow the submucosa to retract and minimize the risk of perforation. In some situations it can be useful to follow the suggestion of Soehendra *et al.* who favor the use of a 0.4 mm monofilament stainless steel wire snare which is pressed firmly against the mucosa to entrap the lesion [36]. A number of braided and barbed snares are now commercially available in different sizes and shapes and can be helpful when removing flat colonic lesions.

The technique described above is also known as submucosal-injection polypectomy or lift and cut mucosal resection and is the most frequently used way of removing early colonic neoplasms regardless of the morphology and the size. For lesions larger than 25 mm, piecemeal resection is invariably required. In the case of piecemeal mucosal resection by using the lift and cut technique, when a portion of a sessile polyp is resected, one edge of the reopened snare can be placed in the divot created by the previous resection so that the same maneuver is repeated on the adjacent portion of polyp, continuing in this manner until resection is complete. In some instances, it may be necessary to change from a jumbo or standard snare to a minisnare to successfully remove smaller fragments at the border of the lesion.

Lesions draped over mucosal folds, extending in a circumferential manner or flat and larger than 30 mm can be a difficult challenge. Additional EMR techniques such as the use of a cap may be required to successfully proceed with endoscopic resection of these lesions. Although most upper gastrointestinal

EMRs in Japan are carried out using the 'suction cap', this technique has proved less popular for colonic EMR.

This is probably due to the perception that the risk of perforation may be greater in the colon than in the stomach. The use of a cap does not increase the difficulty of colonoscopy; it can improve diagnostic yield and can allow more precise targeting of polyps [37].

Nevertheless, considerable skill is required to control suction so as not to aspirate the full thickness of the colonic wall and avoid strangulating the mucosa with the snare too near the base of the created bleb [33,38].

Sadahiro et al. [39] demonstrated, using colorectal cancer surgical specimens, that a cap with a height of 7 mm is more suitable for the colon, while either a 7mm cap or a 10 mm cap could be used in the rectum.

In our experience and in other reported experiences the cap-mucosectomy technique in the colon may add a significant advantage in removing lesions behind mucosal folds, both increasing the visual field and improving the ability to focus the target lesion during resection maneuvers [38,40].

The inject, lift, and cut technique is another modality of performing EMR which uses a double-channeled endoscope. First the lesion is lifted with submucosal injection as described earlier. A snare is then passed through one channel and a forceps through the other. The forceps are used to grasp and lift the lesion allowing it to be ensnared. The use of a double-channel scope in the colon is challenging because of its rigidity, and using the two devices at the same time may be very complicated in the colon where the available operative lumen is much smaller than in the stomach where the technique has been originally described. We have found this technique difficult to perform and not very beneficial and the reported use for colonic lesions is very scarce in the literature. To improve access to mucosal lesions, the use of two endoscopes inserted in parallel has been proposed. One endoscope is then used to lift and manipulate the lesion while the other is used to resect the mucosa with a better ability to identify the dissection line and properly to control the devices used for the endoscopic procedures [41].

Endoscopic submucosal dissection for colonic lesions

For the curative treatment of mucosal colonic lesions, the most important issue is the completeness of the resection. This task can be difficult to achieve in large sessile polyps and residual tumor may be left behind, leading to local recurrence. Conventional techniques of EMR such as the cap assisted, strip biopsy, with ligating device etc., are thought to be inadequate for en bloc resection of large colonic lesions. The multiple fragments that result from this piecemeal resection make the histopathologic evaluation of the completeness of polyp removal difficult.

Therefore, en bloc resection with an adequate tumor cell-negative margin is considered a more desirable outcome. The technical limitations in endoscopic treatment of large colonic lesions can sometimes be overcome by a device enabling the performance of en bloc resection, thus allowing the acquisition of a single large specimen for the correct evaluation of the resection margins.

In 1995 Hosokawa and Yoshida [42] developed a new device for EMR: the insulated-tip electrosurgical knife (It-knife) which has a ceramic bulb at the tip to prevent injury to deeper layers of the GI tract. It was reported that EMR with an It-knife made it possible to perform en bloc resections of large early stage gastric cancers with a reduction in the recurrence rate [43,44].

Subsequently a number of different knives with specific technical peculiarities, such as the hook-knife or the flex-knife have been introduced in clinical practice by Japanese endoscopists with extensive experience in submucosal dissection of early gastric cancer [45].

As for standard colonic EMR, formation of a good submucosal cushion of the targeted mucosa is one of the most important elements for a successful ESD. Because the colonic wall is thinner than the gastric wall, it is more difficult to inject sodium hyaluronate solution or other viscous substances into the appropriate submucosal layer of the colon. To avoid injections of sodium hyaluronate into the wrong layer, pre-injections of small amounts of normal saline into the submucosal layer are useful. By mixing a small amount of indigo carmine dye or methylene blue into the injected solution, the injected area of the sodium can be distinguished much more easily from the non-injected area even after pre-injections of normal saline.

As previously described by a Korean group [46], we are testing in animal studies the possibility of injecting fibrin glue that is able to create a stable and thick cushion and provide an excellent hemostatic effect which can be useful for preventing both intraprocedural and delayed bleeding [47]. Unlike ESD of early gastric cancer, marking placement can be omitted for ESD of colonic neoplastic lesions in the majority of cases because the margins of the lesions are clearly visible even after submucosal injections especially if chromoendoscopy with indigo carmine has been performed prior to resection.

After a sufficient protrusion of the mucosa is produced, a small mucosal incision with a needle knife is created in the two opposite areas of the tumor and thereafter the circumferential mucosal incision with a knife can be performed safely. A cylindric transparent hood, 8 mm in length, or a standard transparent cap, attached to the endoscope tip are also very helpful for the safety of mucosal incision by reducing unintentional movements of the colonic wall toward the needle knife. But this technique is more demanding and is only sporadically used for resection of non-gastric lesions such as large colonic neoplasms [48–50].

The main reasons for the difficulty are the inability to use countertraction for good visualization of the targeted tissue.

With regard to endoscopic submucosal dissection (ESD) into the stomach, scope retroflexion in the colon is one of the most required maneuvers to approach large lesions and especially those located behind folds, on the proximal end of tight turns or involving more than two-thirds of the circumference.

In order to facilitate retroflexion, especially in the left colon, we use a therapeutic gastroscope whose flexibility is greater than a standard colonoscope and allowed to easily retroflex in all the colonic segments. A potential alternative to the therapeutic gastroscope can be a pediatric colonoscope with a short bending section [51], designed to improve therapeutic access in the colon.

Working with the scope retroflexed in the colon does not negatively affect in any instance the ability to maneuver the devices required to complete the submucosal incision including the use of clips or argon plasma coagulation probes.

For the submucosal dissection, a forced coagulation mode of 25 W is selected. The submucosal dissection is progressively performed by advancing the submucosal dissection while sliding the tip of the endoscope with a hood under the dissected mucosa. Effective control of bleeding during the procedure is a key element for a successful ESD. We think that intraprocedural bleeding must be promptly controlled whenever it occurs regardless of its severity. An endoscopic field which is dirty with fresh blood or clots makes it difficult to identify the submucosal resection plane as well as the lesion margin.

During submucosal dissection blood vessels can be recognized during the submucosal incision because it is performed under direct visualization of the tissue. When blood vessels are recognized, the output mode is changed to the argon plasma coagulation mode. Because the voltage of the argon plasma coagulation mode is higher than the coagulation mode, small blood vessels can be cut without bleeding.

Bleeding can also be prevented or stopped by using hemostatic forceps. The generator is set to soft coagulation mode (50–80 W) for hemostatic forceps which are used to pinch a blood vessel precisely, retract it, and coagulate with a minimal contact area.

Perforation is a major concern as a possible complication of ESD. Perforation during ESD using sodium hyaluronate can be minimized by sufficiently thickening the submucosa by proper injection of sodium hyaluronate and careful selection of the layer for incision.

In our experience, the increased risk of wall perforation is due also to the reduced room of colonic lumen and the variety of angles and folds in the colon which make the proper control of knife movements very difficult as it may be challenging to control the depth and the direction of the cut at the same time. The risk can be further increased when the lesion is infiltrating the submucosa and injection cannot adequately create a submucosal cushion. For this reason careful inspection of the submucosal layer during its dissection is required to identify submucosal tissue or irregularities compatible with deep neoplastic invasion.

When a perforation is made during the procedure, it is usually small and recognized immediately; therefore, it can be closed with endoscopic clip placements and can be managed conservatively [35].

Outcome

Endoscopic mucosal resection (EMR) represents a major therapeutic advance in the management of early cancer of the upper and lower gastrointestinal tract. In the colon, lymph node metastasis occurs only after penetration of the submucosa and is directly correlated to the depth of submucosal penetration by the tumor [52]. This supports the therapeutic effectiveness of endoscopic removal of polyps and flat lesions when confined to the mucosa, regardless of their size.

Various studies have been published on the safety and therapeutic potential of EMR for colonic tumors since the first data were reported by Tata et al. in 1984 [53].

Yokota et al. in their series involving 137 flat lesions resected by EMR achieved a complete removal in 87% with complication rates of 0.7% and 0.4% for perforation and bleeding, respectively [54]. Bergmann and Beger used EMR for 71 lesions of sizes ranging from 10 to 50 mm [55]. They encountered one case of bleeding which was treated endoscopically and one case of perforation treated by surgery. At 18 months follow-up local recurrence was observed in two cases. Similar results in terms of technical success (98.1%), complication rate (9.6%), and recurrence rate (15%) have been recently reported by a French group in 50 patients affected by advanced sessile adenoma and early-stage colorectal carcinoma [56].

Sometimes en bloc resection of large sessile polyps is not possible and endoscopic piecemeal mucosal resection is performed. Iishi et al. [57] reported from their study on 42 large polyps that with intense follow-up program piecemeal resection can also be safe and effective.

The proportion of piecemeal vs. en bloc resection seems to be directly correlated with the diameter of the lesions. In a recent paper, despite the use of a long-lasting solution for submucosal injection, the rate of en bloc resection decreased from 85.9% in the case of lesions between 10 mm and 19 mm to 23.1% for lesions between 20 mm and 29 mm [58]. In the study by Su et al., piecemeal resection was invariably required for all colonic flat lesions larger than 30 mm [59].

The appearance of carcinoma after removal of adenomatous polyps is rare. In only one study, published by Walsh et al. [60], carcinoma was reported to have occurred in 5% of patients during follow-up.

Less extensive data have been published on the use of EMR-C for colonic lesions because its application in the colon remains controversial while EMR-C has been used extensively to treat early-stage esophageal and gastric cancers. Tada *et al.* [37] used EMR-C in the colon and achieved full thickness resection of the mucosal layer and a third of the submucosal layer.

In a paper from our group, the EMR-C technique was used with minimal complications in 46 patients [38]. The lack of perforation in these studies can be attributed to the large volume of fluid injected submucosally and the judicious application of suction with the cap. Resection of 10.8% of the polyps was complicated by bleeding, usually larger polyps. In all cases, bleeding was intraprocedural and was easily controlled by endoscopic techniques. Post-polypectomy syndrome with fever and abdominal pain occurred in a few patients.

In the Bergmann series, the EMR-C technique was successfully used only if snare resection was not feasible [55]. It has been suggested that full suction should not be used during EMR-C to avoid grasping of the muscularis propria [60].

Sometimes it may be very challenging to access the target area for EMR when neoplastic disease had migrated proximally beyond the forward-viewing field of the endoscope.

A prospective technical endoscopic evaluation of retroflexion EMR using cap-assisted dissection as a method of luminal 'salvage' therapy was conducted in patients referred to a tertiary endoscopy unit, in whom colonic lesions had been assessed as unresectable using conventional forward-viewing EMR at the index colonoscopy, who were therefore candidates for direct surgical resection. All 68 patients fulfilling the criteria were succesfully treated with success rate, complications, and mid-term recurrence comparable to a previous study of colonic EMR [61]. Retroflexion EMR with a cap may therefore offer 'salvage' endoluminal therapy in patients in whom surgical resection would otherwise have been required.

Overall, whatever the technique used, the two most frequently reported major complications are perforation (0–5%) and bleeding (0.5–6%) and both may be potentially controlled with endoscopic methods and very rarely require surgical treatment (11,62–64).

Removal of large sessile lesions is technically demanding and often requires up to two hours. The length and the difficulty of the procedure are increased by the need to reintroduce the colonoscope to retrieve fragments of lesions after a piecemeal resection in the colorectum. The complete ablation of large adenoma may require from one to five endoscopic sessions. In most recent studies, all lesions are reported as being removed in a single session [11]. When feasible, this eliminates the discomfort and the inconvenience of repeated procedures.

Follow-up is essential because of the risk of recurrence. Aggressive surveillance seems justified, because it has been shown, in an animal model, that residual tumor has a high regrowth rate [65].

Surveillance is devoted to allowing detection of early regrowth, which is more easily treated by APC or standard polypectomy [38].

Therefore, rigorous follow-up is necessary to detect recurrence. However, the strategy for follow-up is unclear at present. Re-examination between one and three months seems mandatory after resection of an early-stage carcinoma. Follow-up colonoscopy should be done at least every three to six months during the first two years after EMR. Some authors have recommended colonoscopy only at one year after en bloc resection, due to the lower risk of recurrence compared with piecemeal resection. However we prefer to carry out a scrupulous surveillance after endoscopic treatment of an early carcinoma (Fig. 9.4).

The recurrence rate after EMR of sessile colorectal polyps ranges from 0% to 40%, but it is difficult to compare the different series because of wide variations in polyp size and length of follow-up. It is likely that patients with larger adenomas are at higher risk for the development of new polyps [66–68].

In our experience, there is a tendency toward an increased risk of recurrence after EMR for polyps larger than 35 mm [35,38].

When remnants of adenoma remain after EMR, APC has been used to reduce the frequency of residual adenoma by 50% [69]. In the study by Zlatanic *et al.*, [70] the recurrence rate after EMR without APC was 100%, as compared with less than 50% of those treated with complementary APC.

Regula *et al.* [71] completely eradicated polyps in 90% of cases when EMR was combined with APC. Others have found APC to be useful, when required, to complete the eradication of adenomatous tissue [72].

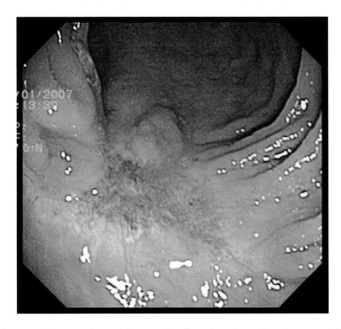

Fig 9.4 Huge scarring area after en bloc resection for a 3 cm large flat adenoma of the rectum.

Nevertheless, in the most recent current studies, EMR has allowed adequate histopathologic assessment of the early colonic neoplasia in all patients, including the identification of invasive cancer [11,12,38]. If EMR is performed properly and all fragments of the polyp are retrieved, the risk of missing a cancer seems negligible.

For this reason, we do not recommend forceps biopsy specimens when a colonic lesion is discovered, provided it is considered, by macroscopic criteria, amenable to EMR.

There are qualitative and quantitative histological features by which nodal involvement may be predicted. A recent study suggested that for tumors without unfavorable histological features such as poor differentiation, vascular invasion, tumor budding, and extensive submucosal invasion (i.e. depth of over 2000 μm from muscularis mucosae or maximum tumor width in the submucosa over 4000 μm), endoscopic resection alone may be considered adequate [73]. Kikuchi *et al.* [74] assessed the risk of recurrence in 17 patients with early stage colorectal cancer infiltrating the upper third of the submucosa. After EMR, there was no local recurrence or lymph node metastasis in any patient. The endoscopic appearance and the characteristics of colonic lesions can usually predict the feasibility and advisability of EMR.

However, if deeper submucosal infiltration is detected in the resection specimens, surgery should be recommended unless operation is precluded by other factors, such as advanced age and/or comorbid disorders.

In conclusion, the ability to retrieve a large resected specimen after EMR allows thorough histopathologic assessment, which can have a significant impact on patient management. The results of the literature data demonstrate that surgery can be avoided for many patients when large colonic lesions are removed by EMR.

Surgical considerations

The use of a laparoscope might be of help in treating colonic polyps or early colonic cancers. Most colonic polyps can be removed during colonoscopy using endoscopic polypectomy. In some patients, however, endoscopic polypectomy or EMR is not possible or is unsafe due to location, size, tortuosity of the colon, adhesions, or complexity of the lesion. In such cases colonoscopic polypectomy or EMR of benign lesions can be performed under laparoscopic guidance.

For laparoscopy-assisted endoscopic polypectomy or EMR, surgeons and monitors are placed according to the segment of colon where the polyp is expected. A 10 mm trocar is inserted for introduction of the videoscope, and two additional trocars are inserted to facilitate the use of additional instruments. The bowel segment is mobilized and the bowel proximal to the polyp-bearing segment is clamped using an atraumatic grasper to prevent distension of the proximal bowel during colonoscopy. This is done because a distended large and small bowel limits laparoscopic visibility.

The colonoscopy should be performed with a minimum of insufflation. Laparoscopic instruments can be used to straighten the bowel to facilitate the advancement of the endoscope. If the lesion is identified, the laparoscopist can present the base of the lesion with laparoscopic graspers for easier snaring by the colonoscopist. When the endoscopic removal of the entire lesions is completed, the extraluminal bowel wall is inspected laparoscopically for signs of transmural involvement of the bowel, either by cautery or by perforation. In case of any suspicion, the defect can be oversewn laparoscopically using seromuscular sutures.

If laparoscopic-assisted colonoscopic polypectomy fails to remove the lesion, alternatives are laparoscopic wedge resection of the polyp or exteriorisation of the affected segment of bowel through a minilaparotomy in order to remove the polyp via colotomy.

The success rate for avoiding a formal bowel resection varies between 67% and 100%. Prohm *et al.* [75] studied six patients with polyps in such unfavorable positions in the rectosigmoid or splenic flexure that they were considered to be more suitable for an open or laparoscopic removal. The polyp-containing segment of the colon was mobilized laparoscopically and stretched as much as possible to facilitate endoscopic polypectomy. No complications occurred. Segmental colectomy was avoided in a series of 12 cases out of 36 patients with problematic adenomas not suitable for endoscopic polypectomy [76]. In another 16 consecutive patients only 40% of the adenomas could be removed by polypectomy under laparoscopic assistance [77].

The removed lesion should undergo immediate frozen section analysis. In the case of malignancy, a laparoscopic bowel resection can be performed immediately according to standard oncological principles.

References

1 Japanese Society for Cancer of the Colon and Rectum. *Japanese Classification of Colorectal Carcinoma*. Kanehara, Tokyo, p. 20, 1997.
2 Hamilton SR, Vogelstein B, Kudo S *et al*. Tumors of the colon and rectum. In: Hamilton SR, & Aaltonen LF, eds. *Pathology and Genetics of Tumors of the Digestive System*. IARC, Lyon, 2000: 103–43.
3 Koyama Y, Kotake K. Overview of colorectal cancer in Japan: report from the Registry of the Japanese Society for Cancer of the Colon and Rectum. *Dis Colon Rectum* 1997; **40** (**10 Suppl**): S2–9.
4 The Paris endoscopic classification of superficial neoplastic lesions: esophagus, stomach, and colon: November 30 to December 1, 2002. *Gastrointest Endosc* 2003; **58**: S3–S43.
5 Churc J, Muto T, Abbau T. Flat lesions of the colorectal mucosa: differences in recognition between American and Japanese endoscopists. *Dis Colon Rectum* 2004; **47**: 1462–6.

6 Muto T, Kamiya J, Sawada T *et al*. Small 'flat adenoma' of the large bowel with special reference to its clinicopathologic features. *Dis Colon Rectum* 1985; **28**: 847–51.

7 Kudo S, Kashida H, Nakajima T *et al*. Endoscopic diagnosis and treatment of early colorectal cancer. *World J Surg* 1997; **21**: 694–701.

8 Ajioka Y, Watanabe H, Kazama S *et al*. Early colorectal cancer with special reference to the superficial non-polypoid type from a histopathologic point of view. *World J Surg* 2000; **24**: 1075–80.

9 Kariya J, Mizuno K, Mayama M. A case of early colonic cancer type IIc associated with familial polyposis coli [in Japanese]. *Stomach Intest* 1977; **12**: 1359–64.

10 Kudo S, Muto T. Superficial depressed type (IIc) of colorectal carcinoma [in Japanese]. *Gastroenterol Endosc* 1986; **28**: 2811–13.

11 Rembacken BJ, Fujii T, Cairns A *et al*. Flat and depressed colonic neoplasms: a prospective study of 1000 colonoscopies in the UK. *Lancet* 2000; **355**: 1211–14.

12 Kudo S, Hashida K. Flat and depressed lesions of the colorectum. *Clin Gastroenterol Hepatol* 2005; **3**: S33–6.

13 Fujimori T, Satonaka K, Yamamura-Idei Y *et al*. Non-involvement of ras mutation on flat colorectal adenomas and carcinomas. *Int J Cancer* 1994; **57**: 51–5.

14 Kudo S. Endoscopic mucosal resection of flat and depressed types of early colorectal cancer. *Endoscopy* 1993; **25**: 455–61.

15 Kudo S. *Early Colorectal Cancer: Detection of Depressed Types of Colorectal Carcinoma*. Igaku-shoin, Tokyo, 1996, pp. 34–6.

16 Hurlstone DP, Sanders DS, Cross SS *et al*. Colonoscopic resection of lateral spreading tumors: a prospective analysis of endoscopic mucosal resection. *Gut* 2004; **53**: 1334–9.

17 Kudo S, Kashida H, Tamura T *et al*. Colonoscopic diagnosis and management of non-polypoid early colorectal cancer. *World J Surg* 2000; **24**: 1081–90.

18 Kudo S. Endoscopic mucosal resection of flat and depressed types of early colorectal cancer. *Endoscopy* 1993; **25**: 455–61.

19 Kudo S, Hirota S, Nakajima T *et al*. Colorectal tumours and pit pattern. *J Clin Pathol* 1994; **47**: 880–5.

20 Kudo S, Rubio CA, Teixeira CR *et al*. Pit pattern in colorectal neoplasia: endoscopic magnifying view. *Endoscopy* 2001; **33**: 367–73.

21 Kashida H, Kudo S. Early colorectal cancer: concept, diagnosis and management. *Int J Clin Oncol* 2006; **11**: 1–8.

22 Kiesslich R, von Bergh M, Hahn M *et al*. Chromoendoscopy with indigocarmine improves the detection of adenomatous and non-adenomatous lesions in the colon. *Endoscopy* 2001; **33**: 1001–6.

23 Harada N, Hamada S, Kubo H *et al*. Preoperative evaluation of submucosal invasive colorectal cancer using a 15-MHz ultrasound miniprobe. *Endoscopy* 2001; **33**: 237–40.

24 Hizawa K, Suekane H, Aoyagi K *et al*. Use of endosonographic evaluation of colorectal tumor depth in determining the appropriateness of endoscopic mucosal resection. *Am J Gastroenterol* 1996; **91**: 768–71.

25 Saitoh Y, Obara T, Einami K *et al*. Efficacy of high-frequency ultrasound probes for the preoperative staging of invasion depth in flat and depressed colorectal tumors. *Gastrointest Endosc* 1996; **44**: 34–9.

26 Uno Y, Munakata A. The non-lifting sign of invasive colon cancer. *Gastrointest Endosc* 1994; **40**: 485–9.

27 Kitamura K, Takahashi T, Yamaguchi T *et al*. Identification, by activated carbon injection, of cancer lesion during laparoscopic surgery. *Lancet* 1994; **343**: 789.

28 Machida H, Sano Y, Hamamoto Y *et al*. Narrow-band imaging in the diagnosis of colorectal mucosal lesions: a pilot study. *Endoscopy* 2004; **36**: 1094–8.

29 Cho E, Uno K, Tanaka K *et al*. Clinical usefulness of endoscopic optimal coherence tomography (EOCT) in the diagnosis of colorectal diseases: a comparative study with EUS using ultrasonic probe. *Gastrointest Endosc* 2003; **57**: T1461.

30 Kiesslich R, Burg J, Vieth M *et al*. Confocal laser endoscopy for diagnosing intraepithelial neoplasias and colorectal cancer in vivo. *Gastroenterology* 2004; **127**: 706–13.

31 Deyle P, Largiader F, Jenny S *et al*. A method for endoscopic electroresection of sessile colonic polyps. *Endoscopy* 1973; **5**: 38–40.

32 Van Gossum A, Cozzoli A, Adler M *et al.* Colonoscopic snare polypectomy: analysis of 1485 resections comparing two types of current. *Gastrointest Endosc* 1992; **38**: 472–5.

33 Conio M, Repici A, Demarquay JF *et al.* EMR of large sessile colorectal polyps. *Gastrointest Endosc* 2004; **60**: 234–41.

34 Inoue H, Takeshita K, Hori H *et al.* Endoscopic mucosal resection with a cap-fitted panendoscope for esophagus, stomach, and colon mucosal lesions. *Gastrointest Endosc* 1993; **39**: 58–62.

35 Repici A, Conio M, De Angelis C *et al.* Insulated-tip knife endoscopic mucosal resection of large colorectal polyps unsuitable for standard polypectomy. *Am J Gastroenterol* 2007; **102**: 1617–23.

36 Soehendra N, Binmoeller KF, Bohnacker S. Endoscopic snare mucosectomy in the esophagus without any additional equipment: a simple technique for resection of flat early cancer. *Endoscopy* 1997; **29**: 380–3.

37 Inoue H, Kawano T, Tani M *et al.* Endoscopic mucosal resection using a cap-technique for use and preventing perforation. *Can J Gastroenterol* 1999; **13**: 477–80.

38 Tada M, Inoue H, Yabata E *et al.* Colonic mucosal resection using a transparent cap-fitted endoscope. *Gastrointest Endosc* 1996; **44**: 63–5.

39 Sadahiro S, Ishida H, Tokunaga N *et al.* Experimental assessment of endoscopic mucosectomy with a cap-fitted panendoscope. *Endoscopy* 1998; **30**: 713–17.

40 Yoshikane H, Hidano H, Sakakibara A *et al.* Efficacy of a distal attachment in endoscopic resection of colorectal polyps situated behind semilunar folds. *Endoscopy* 2001; **33**: 440–2.

41 Brooker JC, Saunders BP, Suzuki N *et al.* Twin-endoscope scissors resection (T-ESR): a new minimally invasive technique for performing colonic mucosectomy. *Surg Endosc* 2001; **15**: 1463–6.

42 Hosokawa K, Yoshida S. Recent advances in endoscopic mucosal resection for early gastric cancer [in Japanese with English abstract]. *Jpn J Cancer Chemother* 1998; **25**: 476–83.

43 Ohkuwa M, Hosokawa N, Boku N *et al.* New endoscopic treatment technique for intratumoural gastric tumours using an insulated-tip diathermic knife. *Endoscopy* 2001; **33**: 221–6.

44 Ono H. Early gastric cancer: diagnosis, pathology, treatment techniques and treatment outcomes. *Eur J Gastroenterol Hepatol* 2006; **18**(8): 863–6.

45 Yamamoto H, Yahagi N, Oyama T. Mucosectomy in the colon with endoscopic submucosal dissection. *Endoscopy* 2005; **37**(8): 764–8.

46 Lee SH, Cho WY, Kim HJ *et al.* A new method of EMR: submucosal injection of a fibrinogen mixture. *Gastrointest Endosc* 2004; **59**: 220–4.

47 Repici A, Sapino A, Preatoni P *et al.* *Endoscopic fibrin glue injection with standard sclerosis needle is effective for submucosal injection before mucosal resection. A comparison test with double channel injector.* Presented at UEGW Berlin, 2006.

48 Gotoda T, Kondo H, Ono H *et al.* A new endoscopic mucosal resection procedure using an insulation-tipped electrosurgical knife for rectal flat lesions. Report of two cases. *Gastrointest Endosc* 1999; **50**: 560–3.

49 Akahoshi K, Kubokawa M, Fujimaru T *et al.* Endoscopic resection of a large pedunculated colonic polyp using an insulated-tip diathermy knife. *Endoscopy* 2005; **37**: 405–6.

50 Fujishiro M, Yahagi N, Nakamura M *et al.* Endoscopic submucosal dissection for rectal epithelial neoplasia. *Endoscopy* 2006; **38**: 493–7.

51 Kessler WR, Rex DK. Impact of bending section length on insertion and retroflexion properties of pediatric and adult colonoscopes. *Am J Gastroenterol* 2005; **100**: 1290–5.

52 Yamamoto S, Watanabe M, Hasegawa H *et al.* The risk of lymph node metastasis in T1 colorectal carcinoma. *Hepatogastroenterology* 2004; **51**: 998–1000.

53 Tada M, Murata M, Murakami F *et al.* Development of the strip-off biopsy [in Japanese]. *Gastroenterol Endosc* 1984; **26**: 833–9.

54 Yokota T, Sugihara K, Yoshida S. Endoscopic mucosal resection for colorectal neoplastic lesions. *Dis Col Rectum* 1994; **37**: 1108–11.

55 Bergmann U, Beger HG. Endoscopic mucosal resection for advanced non-polypoid colorectal adenoma and early stage carcinoma. *Surg Endosc* 2003; **17**: 475–9.

56 Bories E, Pesenti C, Monges G *et al.* Endoscopic mucosal resection for advanced sessile adenoma and early-stage colorectal carcinoma. *Endoscopy* 2006; **38**: 231–5.

57 Iishi H, Tatsuta M, Iseki K *et al.* Endoscopic piecemeal resection with submucosal saline injection of large colorectal polyps. *Gastrointest Endosc* 2000; **51**: 697–700.

58 Katsinelos P, Kountouras J, Paroutoglou G *et al.* Endoscopic mucosal resection of large sessile colorectal polyps with submucosal injection of hypertonic 50 percent dextrose-epinephrine solution. *Dis Colon Rectum* 2006; **49**: 1384–92.

59 Su MY, Hsu CM, Ho YP *et al.* Endoscopic mucosal resection for colonic non-polypoid neoplasms. *Am J Gastroenterol* 2005; **100**: 2174–9.

60 Walsh RM, Ackroyd FW, Shellito PC. Endoscopic resection of large sessile colorectal polyps. *Gastrointest Endosc* 1992; **38**: 303–9.

61 Hurlstone DP, Sanders DS, Thomson M *et al.* 'Salvage' endoscopic mucosal resection in the colon using a retroflexion gastroscope dissection technique: a prospective analysis. *Endoscopy* 2006; **38**: 902–6.

62 Mana F, De Vogelaere K, Urban D. Iatrogenic perforation of the colon during diagnostic colonoscopy: endoscopic treatment with clips. *Gastrointest Endosc* 2001; **54**: 258–9.

63 Matsuda T, Fujii T, Emura F *et al.* Complete closure of large defect after EMR of lateral spreading colorectal tumor when using a two-channel colonoscope. *Gastrointest Endosc* 2004; **57**: 836–8.

64 Hurlstone DP, Lobo AJ. A new technique for endoscopic resection of large lateral spreading tumors of the colon: dual intubation colonoscopy with endoclip-assisted 'loop suturing' method. *Am J Gastroenterol* 2002; **97**: 2931–2.

65 Kunihiro M, Tanaka S, Haruma K *et al.* Electrocautery snare resection stimulates cellular proliferation of residual colorectal tumor: an increasing gene expression related to tumor growth. *Dis Colon Rectum* 2000; **43**: 1107–15.

66 Yoshikane H, Hidano H, Sakakibara A *et al.* Endoscopic resection of laterally spreading tumours of the large intestine using a distal attachment. *Endoscopy* 1999; **31**: 426–30.

67 Bedogni G, Bertoni G, Ricci E *et al.* Colonoscopic excision of large and giant colorectal polyps. Technical implication and result over eight years. *Dis Colon Rectum* 1986; **29**: 831–5.

68 Noshirwani KC, van Stolk RU, Rybicki LA *et al.* Adenoma size and number are predictive of adenoma recurrence: implications for surveillance colonoscopy. *Gastrointest Endosc* 2000; **51**: 433–7.

69 Brooker JC, Saunders BP, Shah SG *et al.* Treatment with argon plasma coagulation reduces recurrence after piecemeal resection of large sessile colonic polyps: a randomized trial and recommendations. *Gastrointest Endosc* 2002; **55**: 371–5.

70 Zlatanic J, Waye JD, Kim PS *et al.* Large sessile colonic adenomas: use of argon plasma coagulator to supplement piecemeal snare polypectomy. *Gastrointest Endosc* 1999; **49**: 731–5.

71 Regula J, Wronska E, Polkowski M *et al.* Argon plasma coagulation after piecemeal polypectomy of sessile colorectal adenomas: long-term follow-up study. *Endoscopy* 2003; **35**: 212–18.

72 Grund KE, Storek D, Farin G. Endoscopic argon plasma coagulation (APC): first clinical experiences in flexible endoscopy. *Endosc Surg Allied Technol* 1994; **2**: 42–4.

73 Ueno H, Mochizuki H, Hashiguchi Y *et al.* Risk factors for an adverse outcome in early invasive colorectal carcinoma. *Gastroenterology* 2004; **127**: 385–94.

74 Kikuchi R, Takano M, Takagi K *et al.* Management of early invasive colorectal cancer. Risk of recurrence and clinical guidelines. *Dis Colon Rectum* 1995; **38**: 1286–95.

75 Prohm P, Weber J, Bonner C. Laparoscopic-assisted coloscopic polypectomy. *Dis Colon Rectum* 2001; **44**: 746–8.

76 Mal F, Perniceni T, Levard H *et al.* Colonic polyps considered unresectable by endoscopy. Removal by combinations of laparoscopy and endoscopy in 65 patients. *Gastroenterol Clin Biol* 1998; **22**: 425–30.

77 Le Picard P, Vacher B, Pouliquen X. Laparoscopy assisted polypectomy or how to be helped by laparoscopy to prevent colectomy in benign polyps considered to be unresectable by colonscopy. *Ann Chir* 1997; **51**: 986–9.

CHAPTER 10

Histopathology of Endoscopic Resection in the Gastrointestinal Tract

MICHAEL VIETH, RALF KIESSLICH, AND KAIYO TAKUBO

Introduction

First, one has to note that the term 'endoscopic mucosal resection' is wrong in respect of anatomical structures because not only the mucosal layer but also preferably most of the submucosal layer should be removed endoscopically in the case of early neoplasia in the gastrointestinal (GI) tract. Therefore, in this chapter the more correct term 'endoscopic resection' (ER) is used. The diagnosis of early cancer in the GI tract has become very important since new endoscopic techniques nowadays allow local endoscopic resections instead of surgical procedures in selected cases. The advantage of surgery is the removal of potentially involved regional lymph nodes. But on the other hand it is known that many patients with early carcinoma will never develop metastases. Patients need to be selected by assessment of high and low risk criteria to offer a local therapy instead of a surgical procedure. Therefore, histopathological evaluation of the resection specimen is very important. In the different parts of the GI tract such as the esophagus, stomach, and colon the risk of lymph node involvement is variable [1–4]. The lowest frequency is given for early colon adenocarcinomas compared to other locations in the GI tract. There are several endoscopic techniques used throughout the GI tract that are described in various chapters of this book.

Gross description and work-up of endoscopic resections

Prior to sending an endoscopic resection specimen to a pathologist some requirements are necessary to achieve the best possible quality of the specimen. From our own experience we know that if you want to preserve fresh material

Endoscopic Mucosal Resection. Edited by M. Conio, P. Siersema, A. Repici and T. Ponchon. © 2008 Blackwell Publishing. ISBN 978-1-4051-5885-5.

the best method to freeze specimens in liquid nitrogen is to embed them completely in 'OCT Cryocompound' (e.g. Leica, Wetzlar, Germany) prior to freezing the specimen. This minimizes freezing artefacts and even allows such specimens to be shipped worldwide in transport containers for liquid nitrogen (e.g. GT series, Air liquide, Kornwestheim, Germany). In the Institute of Pathology, specimens are taken out and one slice is cut from the middle of the specimen without letting the specimen warm up. One frozen section should be performed from this slice to document the content of this material. The remaining specimen will be fixed in formalin as with all ordinary specimens. The advantage of this method is the fresh material that can be used for further analysis. The disadvantage is that specimens cannot be orientated so that the closest margin can be recognized and the specimen orientated respectively.

In respect of quality it is better to receive specimens fixed in formalin. Prior to fixation, specimens in formalin needles should be used either to fix the specimen on cork or on a piece of thick paper. It is very important not to create tension on the specimen because formalin leads to shrinking in about 20% of endoscopic specimens (through fixation small biopsies shrink about 50%). The specimen should be fixed very loosely on the piece of cork in order to take shrinkage into account and avoid tension artefacts due to formalin.

In the Institute of Pathology the specimen is orientated in a manner that the closest margin to the neoplasia can be detected. We use a microscope for reverse light to orientate the specimen at a 20-fold magnification and if this is not possible, to orientate at a 90-fold magnification. Normally, neoplasias show structural changes of the surface such as erosions, marked gyration, polypoid structures, and irregular folds. The vast majority of specimens can be orientated on the basis of these changes. After orientation it might be useful to mark the basal margin with black ink or latex colors but this is open to discussion because it is probably not necessary if the specimen has not been orientated by the endoscopists in a way that a certain clockwise recognition of the resection margins can be achieved.

After orientation and marking of the margins (especially in those cases in which the endoscopist has given the exact clockwise orientation of the resection margins) the specimen needs to be cut into slices (each about 1–1.5 mm thick). In order to receive the best quality (especially if recuts are necessary) do not place more than two slices into one cassette (the optimum would be a single slice only).

The technique of gross description of endoscopic resection specimens does not vary throughout the GI tract but through histological grading. Every specimen has a three-dimensional size; areas of squamous epithelium and irregular areas on the surface should be reported. Line drawings or photographs are helpful.

Technique

The different techniques of endoscopic resection have so far not been evaluated in randomized controlled trials. The reported series were predominately performed in a small number of highly selected patients with relatively short follow-up periods. It is therefore difficult to compare the efficacy and safety between the various methods. The lift and cut technique and the suck and ligate technique were recently investigated in patients with Barrett's high-grade dysplasia or mucosal cancer [5,6]. Endoscopic mucosal resection with cap (EMR-C) has been extensively studied in patients with early squamous carcinoma of the esophagus [7,8].

Endoscopic submucosal dissection (ESD) is a technique developed with the primary aim of obtaining one-piece resection even in large lesions. This procedure involves circumferential cutting of the mucosa surrounding the tumor followed by dissection of the submucosa beneath the lesion [9–13]. The advantage of ESD is that it provides a single specimen which allows a correct histological statement including the resection margins. Additionally the one-piece resection has been proposed as a gold standard of EMR as it reduces the risk of tumor recurrences [14], but this is controversial because in the hands of experienced groups it has been shown that the piecemeal technique also gives an excellent outcome [15]. The disadvantages of the piecemeal technique that have been discussed, i.e. that it is difficult to recognize complete removal histologically, plays a minor role in early neoplasia because remaining nests of neoplasia can also be recognized endoscopically and can be excluded by bioptic control or complete ablation of questionable areas (especially in Barrett's neoplasia).

As well as new endoscopic techniques it should be noted that new molecular methods still do not answer the questions about what is still regenerative and what is already neoplasia, and what is still high-grade intraepithelial neoplasia and what is already invasive carcinoma. The histological diagnosis by an experienced pathologist is still the gold standard in recognition and grading of neoplasia.

In 2000 the World Health Organization (WHO) [16] recommended that the term 'dysplasia' should not be used any more but that 'intraepithelial neoplasia' should be used instead throughout the gastrointestinal tract. The term 'high-grade intraepithelial neoplasia' replaces and includes 'high-grade dysplasia' and 'carcinoma in situ'. Because of the uncritical use of the term 'dysplasia', quite often regenerative changes were mixed up with early neoplastic changes and sometimes the term dysplasia was also used by some authors to indicate early carcinomas [17]. This led to overdiagnosis and underdiagnosis of regenerative and neoplastic lesions with concommittant confusion of endoscopists due to lack of matching of endoscopical and

Table 10.1   Series of patients with low-grade intraepithelial neoplasia in Barrett's esophagus showing the frequency of neoplasia among the study cohort.

Author	Year	Frequency of low-grade dysplasia (%)
Schnell *et al.* [18]	2001	67.2
Sharma *et al.* [42]	2003	25.0
Egger *et al.* [43]	2003	20.2
O'Connor *et al.* [44]	1999	17.6
Fisher *et al.* [45]	2003	13.5
Csendes *et al.* [46]	2002	11.9
Gopal *et al.* [47]	2003	9.7
Conio *et al.* [48]	2003	9.6
Vieth and Stolte [51]	2002	1.1

histological diagnosis. The world record for low-grade dysplasia is nearly 70% within a consecutive series of patients with Barrett's esophagus [18] (see Table 10.1). Obviously in such series overdiagnosis of regenerative changes led to confusion in the literature since most of these authors concluded that low-grade dysplasia does progress to Barrett's carcinoma in a small fraction only so it is no surprise if series are corrupted by overestimation of regenerative changes.

According to the WHO classification invasive adenocarcinoma is diagnosed whenever the tumor invades into the lamina propria or the submucosal layer in the case of colon carcinoma, which leads to different 'artificial' definitions of carcinoma in the upper and lower GI tract. In the upper GI tract the entity of mucosal carcinoma is existing whereas in the colon the diagnosis of carcinoma is only made if the submucosal layer has been invaded. From a biological point of view this artificial border makes little sense because cytological and histological criteria mean that all mutations and changes in the affected cell populations can already be recognized on the mucosal level. On the other hand, in the colon, lymph node metastases never develop if the lesion is limited to the mucosa.

Squamous cell carcinoma of the esophagus

Early squamous cell cancer of the esophagus is divided into mucosal (m1–3) and submucosal (sm1–3) carcinoma. This has been adapted from the Japanese classification of early neoplasia of the esophagus [19]. Instead of the term 'carcinoma in situ' pT1 m1 is used. Infiltration of the tunica propria is labeled as pT1 m2 tumor and invasion into the muscularis mucosa is named pT1 m3 (see Table 10.2). The more invasive the carcinoma, the higher the risk of lymph node metastasis. The decision in favor of a surgical procedure or local

Depth of infiltration	N+ (%)
m1	0.0
m2 u.-3-type	4.8
sm-type	38.4
sm 1	24.1
sm 2	33.6
sm 3	48.4

Table 10.2 Risk of lymph node metastasis in early squamous cell carcinoma of the esophagus (modified after [20]).

m: mucosal; sm: submucosal.

endoscopical therapy mainly depends on the risk of lymph node metastasis that should be lesser than the risk of the surgical procedure [20].

Due to uncertainties between bioptic diagnosis and diagnosis on resection specimens, the Vienna classification was introduced in 1998 at the World Congress of Gastroenterology [21,22]. The Vienna classification groups diagnoses together in five groups in conjunction with a clinical consequence. This leads to a subsequent loosening of the WHO classification of tumors. Fortunately this is without any consequence since cases with high-grade intraepithelial neoplasia and very early (mucosal) carcinoma need the same clinical treatment, and thus a further subdivision has no clinical consequence.

Adenocarcinoma of the distal esophagus

Up until now the morphogenesis of Barrett's mucosa (specialized intestinal metaplasia) is still unsolved. Furthermore, discrepancies between clear segments or tongues of columnar epithelium in the distal esophagus diagnosed endoscopically and the absence of histological confirmation of a Barrett's diagnosis [23] is a confusing issue between gastroenterologists and pathologists. At least it is known that patients with Barrett's esophagus have an up to 30 times elevated risk of developing Barrett's adenocarcinoma compared to a normal population [24]. The individual risk ranges between 0.5% and 1% per year [25] and varies regionally, with higher rates in Scotland compared to other parts of the world [26].

For Barrett's adenocarcinoma it is very important to carry out a risk stratification for the development of regional lymph node metastasis before undertaking further therapy. For the low risk group the following criteria have been established: well or moderately differentiated; no lymphatic vessel permeation; mucosal carcinoma; and size less than 2 cm. All other cases probably have to be regarded as belonging to a high risk group for the development/existence of lymph node metastasis [27]. Whether or not the biological behavior at the front

Table 10.3 Frequency of lymph node metastasis in early Barrett's adenocarcinoma sub-divided between mucosal (pT1m) and submucosal (pT1sm) type (modified after [49,50]).

	Year	pT1m		pT1sm	
		n	N+ (%)	*n*	N+ (%)
Rice [52]	1997	29	3	17	8
Hölscher [53]	1997	10	0	31	16
Ruol [54]	1997	4	0	22	36
van Sandvick [55]	2000	12	0	20	30
Stein [56]	2000	38	0	56	18
Buskens [57]	2004	33	0	42	29
Westerterp [58]	2005	54	2*	65	28
Liu [59]	2005	42	0	76	26
Stein [60]	2005	70	0	87	22
Bollschweiler [61]	2006	14	0	13	41
DeMeester [62]	2006	78	1	48	25

* Mucosal and sm-1 tumors were analysed together as pT1m.

of the invasion needs to be included into such a risk stratification (Stolte, personal communication) should be discussed. Up until now Barrett's neoplasia has been somewhat roughly divided into a mucosal and submucosal type (sm1–3) (Table 10.3), similar to gastric carcinoma. Sm1 level is defined as infiltration lesser than 500 µm in Western countries, whereas in Japan sm1 infiltration is defined as invasion within 200 µm. Very problematic in this respect is the fact that columnar epithelium in the distal esophagus always show a double layer of muscularis mucosae [28]. Thus it is difficult to describe the depth of infiltration in relation to the muscularis mucosae. Our group therefore proposed a new division of the mucosa into different layers (m1–4) (see Fig. 10.1). Even old cases from the archives can be subclassified. A first analysis of the frequency of presence or absence of lymphatic vessel permeation showed a strong relation to the depth of infiltration (see Table 10.4). These results derive from local endoscopic resection specimens published recently [29].

Difficulties in the distinction between high-grade dysplasia and mucosal carcinoma is well documented through the recent version of the WHO classification (Fig. 1.25, p. 23) where a clear invasive adenocarcinoma is depicted but the footnote below the photograph declares that this is 'high-grade intraepithelial neoplasia' in Barrett's esophagus [16].

The question of whether an adenocarcinoma at the gastroesophageal junction derives from the cardia mucosa or on the base of Barrett's mucosa is sometimes difficult to decide. It becomes more probable that Barrett's adenocarcinoma is present when 'regular' Barrett's mucosa is confirmed close to the carcinoma. The WHO classification proposed to diagnose all adenocarcinomas reaching

(a)

(b)

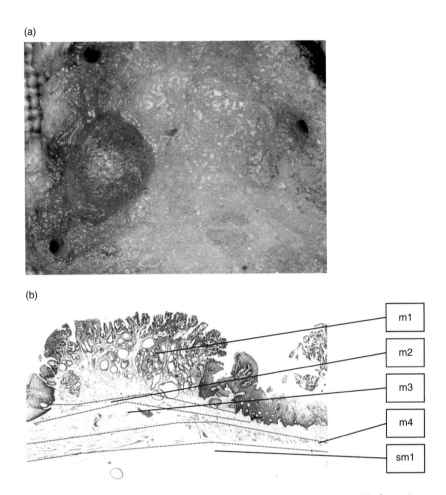

m1

m2

m3

m4

sm1

Fig. 10.1 Mucosal well-differentiated Barrett's adenocarcinoma (m1-type); (a) Endoscopic resection specimen; (b) histopathological section: m2 – infiltration of superficial muscularis mucosae, m3 – infiltration of layer in between superficial and deep muscularis mucosae, m4 – infiltration of deep muscularis mucosae, sm1 – upper third of submucosal layer (<500 μm; or in Japan <200 μm).

the gastroesophageal junction 'tumor of the gastroesophageal junction'. In any case, an etiological diagnosis should preferably always be given. The term 'cardia' should be avoided since no overall and clear anatomic nor histological definition of this region is known. Instead, the term 'proximal gastric carcinoma' should be used. In the case of involvement of the gastroesophageal junction the tumor should be designated as a tumor of the gastroesophageal junction. Squamous cell carcinomas are always excluded [16].

Gastric carcinoma

In 1984 Takaheshi and Iwama [30] showed through three-dimensional reconstruction that lateral fusion and anastomosis with neighboring glands are the

Depth	*n*	L1
Barrett-Ca pT1		
m1	116	1 (0.8%)
m2	37	–
m3	19	–
m4	35	1 (2.8%)

Table 10.4 Frequency of lymphatic vessel permeation in endoscopic resection specimens of mucosal Barrett's adenocarcinoma depending on the depth of infiltration (modified after [49]).

Depth: depth of infiltration; *n*: number of cases; L1: lymphatic permeation of tumor).

first signs of early invasion into the tunica propria. The diagnosis of mucosal carcinoma is possible even without the presence of single tumor cells that are frequently seen in poorly differentiated carcinomas but not in well-differentiated carcinomas.

Worldwide differences in the diagnostic criteria of mucosal carcinomas mostly apply to bioptic diagnoses but not to (endoscopic) resection specimens and are probably just a sign of uncertainty [21,22,31,32] rather than an expression of Japanese or Western viewpoints. Furthermore, due to forensic reasons some pathologists prefer the term 'high-grade intraepithelial neoplasia' rather than adenocarcinoma.

In the literature, follow-up studies on high-grade intraepithelial neoplasia up until the development of invasive gastric adenocarcinoma [32–38] show that within a few months invasive carcinoma is present. This could have led to the speculation that all these cases of carcinoma were already present at the time of bioptic diagnosis but uncertainty led to the histological diagnosis of high-grade dysplasia (intraepithelial neoplasia).

Gastric carcinomas are subdivided into carcinomas of the mucosal layer (m-type) and submucosal layer (sm1–3) (see Table 10.5).

Colon carcinoma

According to national cancer registries colon cancer is by far the most common GI cancer in Europe; the second most common is gastric cancer, and the third most frequent are neoplasms of the esophagus. National data from the German cancer registry show that colon cancer is almost three times more frequent than gastric cancer, and esophageal cancer sums up to less than 10% of the cases of colon cancer [39,40]. Therefore, endoscopic techniques are widely used for colon neoplasms. Fortunately most cases with intraepithelial neoplasia (adenoma) as a precursor for invasive carcinoma are resected. For the decision about endosocopic resection versus surgical treatment, histology needs to distinguish between high and low risk criteria for the presence of regional lymph

Table 10.5 Frequency of lymph node metastasis in gastric carcinoma divided into mucosal (m-) and submucosal (sm-) type (modified after [20]).

Depth of infiltration	N+ (%)
m-type	2.3
sm-type	18.0
sm 1	6.9
sm 2	16.2
sm 3	25.9

m: mucosal; sm: submucosal.

node metasasis (see Table 10.6). Low risk criteria are: depth of infiltration confined to the upper third (1000 µm) or middle third of the submucosal layer; well or moderately differentiated: absence of lymphatic vessel permeation; and absence or slight tumor cell budding at the front of invasion [41]. Poor differentiation, infiltration into the lower third of the submucosal layer (sm3), incomplete resection, presence of lymphatic vessel permeation, and moderate or marked budding of tumor cells are considered as high risk criteria. Venous invasion need not be considered as a risk factor for lymph node metastasis, but for distant hematogenous metastasis that cannot be influenced by surgical treatment. On the other hand it can be discussed that cases with venous invasion might represent cases with higher concomitant risk for lymphatic permeation. But in general, venous invasion is not a factor influencing high or low risk assessment.

Summary

Endoscopic resection techniques for early neoplasms of the gastrointestinal tract need an exact description of the depth of infiltration before the decision is taken about whether to use endoscopic therapy or surgical therapy and before grouping patients into low risk or high risk groups. Histologically, subdivision of the mucosa in early esophageal neoplasms does make sense since the risk of lymph node metastasis increases with the depth of infiltration. Differences between squamous cell carcinoma and adenocarcinoma of the esophagus should be noted.

The distinction of high-grade intraepithelial neoplasia and mucosal carcinoma is almost without further clinical consequence since the diagnosis of high-grade intraepithelial neoplasia should (after clinical staging) at least lead to diagnostic endoscopic resection. The final histological diagnosis could then be made on the resection specimen. Diagnosis of low-grade intraepithelial neoplasia should not be mixed up with regenerative changes. Worldwide criteria on bioptic specimens for intraepithelial neoplasia and invasive carcinoma should be improved further.

Table 10.6 Risk of lymph node metastasis in colon adenocarcinoma subdivided into cases with low and high risk criteria (modified after [41]).

Author	*n*	N+ high risk (%)	N+ low risk (%)
Tanaka *et al.*, 1995 [63]	65	5/42 (11.9)	1/23 (4.3)
Kikuchi *et al.*, 1995 [64]	182	9/36 (25)	4/146 (2.7)
Nivatvongs *et al.*, 1991 [65]	151	13/113 (11.5)	0/38
Jung *et al.*, 1988 [66]	87	1/17 (5.8)	0/70
Hackelsberger *et al.*, 1995 [67]	86	1/45 (2.2)	1/41 (2.4)
Huddy *et al.*, 1993 [68]	27	3/17 (17.6)	0/10
Christie *et al.*, 1988 [69]	101	1/55 (1.8)	0/46
Coverlizza *et al.*, 1989 [70]	81	5/14 (35.7)	0/67
Morson *et al.*, 1984 [71]	60	0/14	0/46
Sugihara *et al.*, 1988 [72]	25	1/18 (5.5)	0/10
Muto *et al.*, 1991 [73]	27	3/20 (15)	0/7
Hermanek 1991 [74]	82	11/41 (27)	2/41 (5)
Stolte, 1991 [75]	60	5/18 (27)	2/42 (5)
Kudo *et al.*, 1993 [76]	80	3/31 (9.6)	0/49
Hase *et al.*, 1995 [77]	79	11/47 (23.4)	0/32
Masaki *et al.*, 2000 [78]	57	2/19 (10.5)	0/38
Schmitt, 2001 [79]	162	17/79 (21.5)	1/83 (1.25)
Moreira *et al.*, 1992 [80]	24	1/13 (7.7)	0/11

References

1 Haggitt RC, Glotzbach RE, Soffer EE, Wruble LD. Prognostic factors in colorectal carcinomas arising in adenomas: implications for lesions removed by endoscopic polypectomy. *Gastroenterology* 1985; **89**: 328–36.
2 Isono K, Sato H, Nakayama K. Results of a nationwide study on the three-field lymph node dissection of esophageal cancer. *Oncology* 1991; **48**: 411–20.
3 Sano T, Kobori O, Muto T. Lymph node metastasis from early gastric cancer: endoscopic resection of tumour. *Br J Surg* 1992; **79**: 241–4.
4 Triantafillidis JK, Cheracakis P. Diagnostic evaluation of patients with early gastric cancer – a literature review. *Hepatogastroenterology* 2004; **51**: 618–24.
5 Nijhawan PK, Wang KW. Endoscopic mucosal resection for lesions with endoscopic features suggestive of malignancy and high-grade dysplasia within Barrett's esophagus. *Gastrointest Endosc* 2000; **52**: 328–32.
6 Ell C, May A, Gossner L et al. Endoscopic mucosal resection of early cancer and high-grade dysplasia in Barrett's esophagus. *Gastroenterology* 2000; **118**: 670–7.
7 Inoue H. Endoscopic mucosal resection for esophageal and gastric mucosal cancers. *Can J Gastroenterol* 1998; **12**: 355–9.
8 Pech O, Gossner L, May A et al. Long-term results of photodynamic therapy with 5-aminolevulinic acid of superficial Barrett's cancer and high-grade intraepithelial neoplasia. *Gastrointest Endosc* 2005; **62**: 24–30.
9 Deinert K, Schumacher B, Preiss C, Stolte M, Neuhaus H. Endoscopic mucosal resection (EMR) as a potentially curative treatment of early neoplasia in Barrett's esophagus. *Gastrointest Endosc* 2005; **61**(5): AB104.
10 Ono H, Kondo H, Gotoda T et al. Endoscopic mucosal resection for treatment of early gastric cancer. *Gut* 2001; **48**: 225–9.

11 Yamamoto H, Yube T, Isoda N et al. A novel method of endoscopic mucosal resection using sodium hyaluronate. *Gastrointest Endosc* 1999; **50**: 251–6.

12 Miyamoto S, Muto M, Hamamoto Y et al. A new technique for endoscopic mucosal resection with an insulated tip electrosurgical knife improves the completeness of resection of intramucosal gastric neoplasms. *Gastrointest Endosc* 2002; **55**: 576–81.

13 Yahagi N, Fujishiro M, Kakushima et al. Endoscopic submucosal dissection for early gastric cancer using the tip of an electro-surgical snare. *Dig Endosc* 2004; **16**: 34–8.

14 Eguchi T, Gotoda T, Oda I et al. Is endoscopic one-piece mucosal resection essential for early gastric cancer? *Dig Endosc* 2003; **15**: 113–16.

15 Seewald S, Akaraviputh T, Seitz U et al. Circumferential EMR and complete removal of Barrett's epithelium: a new approach to management of Barrett's esophagus containing high-grade intraepithelial neoplasia and intramucosal carcinoma. *Gastrointest Endosc* 2003; **57**: 854–9.

16 WHO classification. (2000) *Tumours of the Digestive System.* Hamilton R and Aaltonen LA, eds. IARC Press, Lyon, 2000.

17 Lewin KJ, Appelman HD. Tumors of the esophagus and stomach. Fascicle 18 of third series. In: *Atlas of Tumor Pathology.* Armed Forces Institute of Pathology, Washington 1995.

18 Schnell TG, Sontag SJ, Chejfec G et al. Long-term nonsurgical management of Barrett's esophagus with high-grade dysplasia. *Gastroenterology* 2001; **120**: 1607–19.

19 Endo M, Kawano T. Detection and classification of early squamous cell esophageal cancer. *Dis Esophagus* 1997; **10**: 155–8.

20 Langner C, Denk H. Meta-analysis of frequency of lymph node metastasis of early gastrointestinal carcinoma. *Verh Dtsch Ges Path* 2003; **87**: 254–6.

21 Schlemper RJ, Dawsey SM, Itabashi M et al. Differences in the diagnostic criteria for esophageal squamous cell carcinoma between Japanese and Western pathologists. *Cancer* 2000; **88**: 996–1006.

22 Schlemper RJ, Riddell RH, Kato Y et al. The Vienna classification of gastrointestinal epithelial neoplasia. *Gut* 2000; **47**: 251–5.

23 Armstrong D. Review article: towards consistency in the endoscopic diagnosis of Barrett's oesophagus and columnar metaplasia. *Aliment Pharmacol Ther* 2004; **Suppl 5**: 40–7.

24 Solaymani-Dodaran M, Logan RF, West J, Card T, Coupland C. Risk of oesophageal cancer in Barrett's oesophagus and gastro-oesophageal reflux. *Gut* 2004; **53**: 1070–4.

25 Shaheen N. Is there a "Barrett's iceberg?". *Gastroenterology* 2002; **123**: 636–9.

26 Jankowski JA, Provenzale D, Moayyedi P. Esophageal adenocarcinoma arising from Barrett's metaplasia has regional variations in the West. *Gastroenterology* 2002; **122**: 588–90.

27 Pech O, May A, Gossner L, Rabenstein T, Ell C. Management of pre-malignant and malignant lesions by endoscopic resection. *Best Pract Res Clin Gastroenterol* 2004; **18**: 61–76.

28 Takubo K, Sasajima K, Yamashita K, Tanaka Y, Fujita K. Double muscularis mucosae in Barrett's esophagus. *Hum Pathol* 1991; **22**: 1158–61.

29 Vieth M, Ell C, Gossner L, May A, Stolte M. Histological analysis of endoscopic resection specimens from 326 patients with Barrett's esophagus and early neoplasia. *Endoscopy* 2004; **36**: 776–81.

30 Takahashi T, Iwama N. Architectural pattern of gastric adenocarcinoma – a 3-dimensional reconstruction study. *Virchows Arch A Pathol Anat Histopathol* 1984; **403**: 127–34.

31 Stolte M. Diagnosis of gastric carcinoma: Japanese fairy tales or Western deficiency? *Virchows Arch* 1999; **434**: 279–80.

32 Stolte M. The new Vienna classification of epithelial neoplasia of the gastrointestinal tract: advantages and disadvantages. *Virchows Arch* 2003; **442**: 99–106.

33 Lansdown M, Quirke P, Dixon MF, Axon AT, Johnston D. High grade dysplasia of the gastric mucosa: a marker for gastric carcinoma. *Gut* 1990; **31**: 977–83.

34 Rugge M, Farinati F, Di Mario F, Baffa R, Valiante F, Cardin F. Gastric epithelial dysplasia: a prospective multicenter follow-up study from the Interdisciplinary Group on Gastric Epithelial Dysplasia. *Hum Pathol* 1991; **22**: 1002–8.

35 Fertitta AM, Comin U, Terruzzi V et al. Clinical significance of gastric dysplasia: a multicenter follow-up study. Gastrointestinal Endoscopic Pathology Study Group. *Endoscopy* 1993; **25**: 265–8.

36 Di Gregorio C, Morandi P, Fante R, De Gaetani C. Gastric dysplasia. A follow-up study. *Am J Gastroenterol* 1993; **88**: 1714–19.

37 Rugge M, Farinati F, Baffa R *et al.* Gastric epithelial dysplasia in the natural history of gastric cancer: a multicenter prospective follow-up study. Interdisciplinary Group on Gastric Epithelial Dysplasia. *Gastroenterology* 1994; **107**: 1288–96.

38 Kokkola A, Haapiainen R, Laxen F, Puolakkainen P, Kivilaakso E, Virtamo J, Sipponen P. Risk of gastric carcinoma in patients with mucosal dysplasia associated with atrophic gastritis: a follow up study. *J Clin Pathol* 1996; **49**: 979–84.

39 Borchard F. Forms and nomenclature of gastrointestinal epithelial expansion: what is invasion? *Verh Dtsch Ges Path* 2000; **84**; 50–61.

40 Krebs in Deutschland. (2004) *Trends und Häufigkeiten. Arbeitsgemeinschaft bevölkerungs-bezogener Krebsregister.* Robert-Koch-Institut (ed). 4th edn, Saarbrücken, 2004.

41 Deinlein P, Reulbach U, Stolte M, Vieth M. Risk factors for lymphatic metastasis from pT1 colorectal adenocarcinoma. *Pathologe* 2003; **24**: 387–93.

42 Sharma P, Weston AP, Topalovski M, Cherian R, Bhattacharyya A, Sampliner RE. Magnification chromoendoscopy for the detection of intestinal metaplasia and dysplasia in Barrett's oesophagus. *Gut* 2003; **52**: 24–7.

43 Egger K, Werner M, Meining A *et al.* Biopsy surveillance is still necessary in patients with Barrett's oesophagus despite new endoscopic imaging techniques. *Gut* 2003; **52**: 18–23.

44 O'Connor JB, Falk GW, Richter JE. The incidence of adenocarcinoma and dysplasia in Barrett's esophagus: report on the Cleveland Clinic Barrett's Esophagus Registry. *Am J Gastroenterol* 1999; **94**: 2037–42.

45 Fisher RS, Bromer MQ, Thomas RM *et al.* Predictors of recurrent specialized intestinal metaplasia after complete laser ablation. *Am J Gastroenterol* 2003; **98**: 1945–51.

46 Csendes A, Smok G, Burdiles P, Braghetto I, Castro C, Korn O. Effect of duodenal diversion on low-grade dysplasia in patients with Barrett's esophagus: analysis of 37 patients. *J Gastrointest Surg* 2002; **6**: 645–52.

47 Gopal DV, Lieberman DA, Magaret N *et al.* Risk factors for dysplasia in patients with Barrett's esophagus (BE): results from a multicenter consortium. *Dig Dis Sci* 2003; **48**: 1537–41.

48 Conio M, Blanchi S, Lapertosa G *et al.* Long-term endoscopic surveillance of patients with Barrett's esophagus. Incidence of dysplasia and adenocarcinoma: a prospective study. *Am J Gastroenterol* 2003; **98**: 1931–9.

49 Vieth M, Stolte M. Pathology of early gastrointestinal neoplasia. *Best Pract Res Clin Gastroenterol* 2005; **19**: 857–69.

50 Vieth M, Rösch T. Endoscopic mucosal resection and the risk of lymph-node metastases: indications revisited? *Endoscopy* 2006; **38**: 175–9.

51 Vieth M, Stolte M. Barrett's esophagus and neoplasia: data from the Bayreuth Barrett's archive. *Gastroenterology* 2002; **122**: 590–1.

52 Rice TW, Zuccaro G Jr, Adelstein DJ, Rybicki LA, Blackstone EH, Goldblum JR. Esophageal carcinoma: depth of tumor invasion is predictive of regional lymph node status. *Ann Thorac Surg* 1998; **65**: 787–92.

53 Hölscher AH, Bollschweiler E, Schneider PM, Siewert JR. Early adenocarcinoma in Barrett's oesophagus. *Br J Surg* 1997; **84**: 1470–3.

54 Ruol A, Merigliano S, Baldan N *et al.* Prevalence, management and outcome of early adenocarcinoma (pT1) of the esophago-gastric junction. Comparison between early cancer in Barrett's esophagus (type I) and early cancer of the cardia (type II). *Dis Esophagus* 1997; **10**: 190–5.

55 van Sandick JW, van Lanschot JJ, ten Kate FJ *et al.* Pathology of early invasive adenocarcinoma of the esophagus or esophagogastric junction: implications for therapeutic decision making. *Cancer* 2000; **88**: 2429–37.

56 Stein HJ, Feith M, Mueller J, Werner M, Siewert JR. Limited resection for early adenocarcinoma in Barrett's esophagus. *Ann Surg* 2000; **232**: 733–42.

57 Buskens CJ, Westerterp M, Lagarde SM, Bergman JJ, ten Kate FJ, van Lanschot JJ. Prediction of appropriateness of local endoscopic treatment for high-grade dysplasia and early adenocarcinoma by EUS and histopathologic features. *Gastrointest Endosc* 2004; **60**: 703–10.

58 Westerterp M, Koppert LB, Buskens CJ *et al.* Outcome of surgical treatment for early adenocarcinoma of the esophagus or gastro-esophageal junction. *Virchows Arch* 2005; **446**: 497–504.

59 Liu L, Hofstetter WL, Rashid A *et al.* Significance of the depth of tumor invasion and lymph node metastasis in superficially invasive (T1) esophageal adenocarcinoma. *Am J Surg Pathol* 2005; **29**: 1079–85.

60 Stein HJ, von Rahden BH, Feith M. Surgery for early stage esophageal adenocarcinoma. *J Surg Oncol* 2005; **92**: 210–7.

61 Bollschweiler E, Baldus SE, Schröder W, Schneider PM, Hölscher AH. Staging of esophageal carcinoma: length of tumor and number of involved regional lymph nodes. Are these independent prognostic factors? *J Surg Oncol* 2006; **94**: 355–63.

62 DeMeester SR. Adenocarcinoma of the esophagus and cardia: a review of the disease and its treatment. *Ann Surg Oncol* 2006; **13**: 12–30.

63 Tanaka S, Haruma K, Teixeira CR *et al.* Endoscopic treatment of submucosal invasive colorectal carcinoma with special reference to risk factors for lymph node metastasis. *J Gastroenterol* 1995; **30**: 710–7.

64 Kikuchi R, Takano M, Takagi K *et al.* Management of early invasive colorectal cancer. Risk of recurrence and clinical guidelines. *Dis Colon Rectum* 1995; **38**: 1286–95.

65 Nivatvongs S, Rojanasakul A, Reiman HM *et al.* The risk of lymph node metastasis in colorectal polyps with invasive adenocarcinoma. *Dis Colon Rectum* 1991; **34**: 323–8.

66 Jung M, Meier HJ, Mennicken C, Barth HO, Manegold BC. Endoscopic and surgical therapy of malignant colorectal polyps. *Z Gastroenterol* 1988; **26**: 179–84.

67 Hackelsberger A, Fruhmorgen P, Weiler H, Heller T, Seeliger H, Junghanns K. Endoscopic polypectomy and management of colorectal adenomas with invasive carcinoma. *Endoscopy* 1995; **27**: 153–8.

68 Huddy SP, Husband EM, Cook MG, Gibbs NM, Marks CG, Heald RJ. Lymph node metastases in early rectal cancer. *Br J Surg* 1993; **80**: 1457–8.

69 Christie JP. Malignant colon polyps–cure by colonoscopy or colectomy? *Am J Gastroenterol* 1984; **79**: 543–7.

70 Coverlizza S, Risio M, Ferrari A, Fenoglio-Preiser CM, Rossini FP. Colorectal adenomas containing invasive carcinoma. Pathologic assessment of lymph node metastatic potential. *Cancer* 1989; **64**: 1937–47.

71 Morson BC, Whiteway JE, Jones EA, Macrae FA, Williams CB. Histopathology and prognosis of malignant colorectal polyps treated by endoscopic polypectomy. *Gut* 1984; **25**: 437–44.

72 Sugihara K, Muto T, Morioka Y. Management of patients with invasive carcinoma removed by colonoscopic polypectomy. *Dis Colon Rectu* 1989; **32**: 829–34.

73 Muto T, Sawada T, Sugihara K. Treatment of carcinoma in adenomas. *World J Surg* 1991; **15**: 35–40.

74 Hermanek P. Prognosis of colorectal cancers. *Fortschr Med* 1991; **109**: 187–8.

75 Stolte M, Hermanek P. Malignant polyps-pathological factors governing clinical management. In: Williams GT, ed. *Gastrointestinal pathology, current topics in pathology.* Springer, Berlin, Heidelberg, New York, 1990: 277–93.

76 Kudo S. Endoscopical mucosal resection of flat and depressed types of early colorectal cancer. *Endoscopy* 1993; **25**: 455–61.

77 Hase K, Shatney CH, Mochizuki H *et al.* Long-term results of curative resection of "minimally invasive" colorectal cancer. *Dis Colon Rectum* 1995; **38**: 19–26.

78 Masaki T, Muto T. Predictive value of histology at the invasive margin in the prognosis of early invasive colorectal carcinoma. *J Gastroenterol* 2000; **35**: 195–200.

79 Schmitt W, Gospos J, Heid T *et al.* Wide-based, flat and depressed colorectal neoplasia: detection, biological qualities and therapy. *Dtsch Med Wochenschr* 2003; **128 Suppl 2**: S136–8.

80 Moreira LF, Iwagaki H, Inoguchi K, Hizuta A, Sakagami K, Orita K. Assessment of lymph node metastasis and vessel invasion in early rectal cancer. *Acta Med Okayama* 1992; **46**: 7–10.

CHAPTER 11

Follow-up after Endoscopic Mucosal Resection

MIHAI CIOCIRLAN AND THIERRY PONCHON

Principles

Endoscopic mucosal resection (EMR) is used as a diagnostic and therapeutic tool for epithelial lesions of the digestive tract (benign, early stage and advanced adenocarcinoma) as well as for subepithelial lesions. EMR cannot be considered as a definitive diagnostic tool or a definitive treatment, but the major component of a therapy which requires a strict follow-up of the patients.

Benign epithelial lesions

Treatment of benign epithelial lesions is motivated by the risk of already existing malignant foci in the lesion or by the risk of malignant development in time or when lesions are clinically manifest. The prototypes of these lesions are adenomas.

Early stage epithelial cancer

EMR appeared first as a diagnostic tool and is used currently as a curative therapy for early digestive cancer. Therapeutic EMR should have a cost-benefit ratio superior to any other treatment option, usually surgery.

(a) Curative intent EMR (standard indications)
With standard indications, the risk of distant metastases is zero and EMR may be considered curative. Endoscopic follow-up looks for residual tissue in order to confirm that all identifiable neoplastic tissues were removed and detects neoplastic tissue in a curable stage as local recurrence and/or metachronous lesions. Risk factors must be identified in order to better target the follow-up protocol and allow risk modification strategies.

Endoscopic Mucosal Resection. Edited by M. Conio, P. Searsema, A. Repici and T. Ponchon. © 2008 Blackwell Publishing. ISBN 978-1-4051-5885-5.

At present there is no randomized controlled study between a non-follow-up policy and/or between different follow-up timetables. With the exception of colorectal epithelial lesions, follow-up frequency was empirically chosen.

(b) Best cost-efficacy EMR (extended indications)
EMR indications may be extended thus increasing the risk of distant metastases. In this instance, EMR may be the best therapeutic option for patients with high surgical morbidity and mortality. In addition to endoscopic follow-up, an extra digestive follow-up may be indicated to look for these distant metastases. The goal is to find them in curable stages by other therapeutic measures: surgery, chemo-radiotherapy, and so on.

Advanced epithelial cancer

EMR for such lesions is performed with palliative intent, in order to achieve better quality of life. Patients are followed up using clinical and biological parameters.

Esophagus

Early stage adenocarcinoma and high-grade dysplasia (HGD) on Barrett's esophagus

High-grade dysplasia and early mucosal adenocarcinoma are considered standard indications.

Literature survey

Distant recurrences
In surgical series, for mucosal lesions, the risk of distant metastasis was from 0% to 2%. In EMR series, there were no distant metastases when high-grade dysplasia or early adenocarcinomas limited to the mucosa were considered as indications.

Residual tissue
Residual tissue has not been regarded as a failure of EMR, as the lesion may be removed in one or multiple sessions.

Local recurrence
In published series, local recurrence rate was about 7% after 33 months, while after circumferential Barrett resection by EMR was 0–11%. All local recurrences were treatable by repeated EMR.

Risk factors for local recurrence included resection completeness which depends on the lesion size, technique and number of EMR pieces.

Metachronous lesions

Metachronous lesions occurred in 3–5% after 25–33 months respectively. That means that when a first area of high-grade dysplasia has appeared and has been treated, the risk that a second dysplastic areas appears is higher than during the follow-up of a nondysplastic Barrett. Furthermore, this second area could have been missed initially. There were no metachronous lesions when the entire Barrett mucosa was resected [1,2].

Follow-up technique and schedules

Follow-up with endoscopy plus biopsies of all visible lesions has been systematically performed. Some series included high resolution endoscopy, systematic biopsies of the EMR site, four quadrant biopsies of the Barrett mucosa and Lugol chromoscopy if the Barrett mucosa has been removed to verify squamous re-epithelialization [1,2].

In these series, the follow-up was organized at one month, every three months during the first year then every six months or less frequent with a 3-, 6-, and 12-month schedule, then yearly. The follow-up was continued for five years.

Extra digestive surveillance was proposed – transabdominal ultrasonography, endoscopic ultrasound (EUS) and CT scan every three to six months at least during the first year or as long as the follow-up continued.

Risk groups

No risk groups were identified for local recurrence or metachronous lesions.

Risk modification

Removing all Barrett mucosa may protect against local recurrence or metachronous lesions. However, the only two studies published did not confirm this hypothesis, as the first study by Seewald *et al.* [1] did not have any local recurrence or metachronous lesion, after a median follow-up of nine months, while in the second study by Giovannini *et al.* [2], there were two local recurrences in 18 patients after a median follow-up of 18 months.

Inadequate acid suppression post-EMR does not predict local recurrence.

Summary of evidence and recommendations

Early one- to three- month follow-up and repeated EMR is recommended until there is complete local remission. When a complete local remission is obtained, follow-up is done at three and six months during the first year and between

6 and 12 months after the first year. There is no evidence that shorter intervals would be of benefit as all detected lesions were in curable stages by repeated EMR.

Until there is definite proof of risk modification, surveillance of patients with complete ablation of Barrett mucosa is to be done. For patients with Barrett's esophagus, an 1-cm interval four quadrant biopsy protocol at every follow-up ensures detection of metachronous lesions. Chromoscopy is to be performed in order to better target the biopsies.

Even if there are no distant recurrences in EMR series at present and the risk is estimated to be near zero from surgical series, we find that extra-digestive follow-up is necessary, at least in patients with m3/sm lesions, especially using EUS.

Early stage squamous-cell carcinoma and squamous-cell dysplasia

Therapeutic curative EMR may be indicated for squamous cell dysplasia or carcinoma limited to the epithelium or lamina propria (m1, m2), when the risk of distant metastases is zero. Extended indications may include m3 and sm1 lesions.

Literature survey

Distant recurrences
The risk of distant recurrences is zero for carcinoma limited to m1 and m2; 8% for m3 and sm1.

Distant recurrences usually caused the death of the patients: there was one pulmonary metastasis in 82 patients with mucosal and submucosal carcinomas [3], two pulmonary and mediastinal lymph node metastases in 26 patients with m3 and sm1 carcinomas [4], two lymph node metastases in 62 patients with high-grade dysplasia and mucosal carcinomas [5], two out of three lymph node metastases in 62 patients with mucosal and sm1 carcinomas, initially treated by chemo-radiotherapy but with subsequent relapse [6].

Residual tissue
Residual tissue was either considered a signal that EMR should be repeated or it was reported together with local recurrences.

Local recurrence
Local recurrence rate varied from 0% to 31%, depending on parietal invasion.

Risk factors for local recurrences were heterogeneous Lugol staining pattern or multiple synchronous lesions [5,7,8]. Features that influence resection completeness such as piecemeal resection or large lesion diameter were also risk factors. More invasive lesions had increased risk for local recurrence.

Local recurrences were usually treatable by repeated EMR/laser/argon plasma coagulation (APC) or surgery/chemo-radiotherapy in a few cases of submucosal involvement. Local recurrences rarely caused the death of the patient: two advanced carcinomas of eight local recurrences considered unsuitable for treatment due to concomitant comorbidities [7], one invasive carcinoma out of 14 local recurrences treated by radiotherapy complicated by perforation [6].

Metachronous lesions
The incidence of metachronous lesions varied from 0% to 20%, all curable by repeated EMR.

Lugol chromoscopy scattered pattern was a risk factor for metachronous lesion development.

Follow-up technique and schedules
Early follow-up was performed at day one to four post-EMR to check for residual tissue; if found, this was treated by laser/APC [5,6] or EMR sessions were scheduled at one- to three-month intervals. After complete local remission, follow-up continued at three to six months during the first year then at 6–12 months, with Lugol and biopsies.

Two studies with six-month screening intervals during the first year and then annually, found that sometimes local recurrences were advanced and caused the death of the patients [6,7]. On the other hand one study with smaller follow-up intervals – at three months during the first year then at six months – found that all local recurrences were curable by EMR [5].

Extra-esophageal follow-up was proposed to look for distant recurrences by CT scan, ultrasound and endoscopic ultrasound yearly or at six months during the first two years then annually. This was mostly ineffective: either there were no distant recurrences or these were not curable and caused death when found – seven of eight distant recurrences from four series with 232 patients (only three treated by chemo-radiotherapy with two relapses and death) [3–6]. In one paper, a lymph node metastasis untreatable by chemo-radiotherapy was diagnosed after more than one year since the last follow-up, due to non-compliance of the patient [4].

Risk groups
Stratified extra-esophageal surveillance was applied by Esaki *et al.* [6] for patients with significant risk of distant metastases (patients with m3 or sm1 carcinoma).

Risk modification

Soon after EMR, APC/laser was used to treat residual tissue [6], but it did not significantly decrease the rate of local recurrence. Chemo-radiotherapy post-EMR was proposed not only for deep submucosal but also for m3/sm1 carcinomas, with no recurrence or distant metastasis.

Summary of evidence and recommendations

Post-EMR early APC/laser application is not useful for local recurrence prevention. Endoscopic follow-up with Lugol is mandatory because it can detect most local recurrences and all metachronous lesions in early curable stages by EMR. Shorter follow-up intervals are probably better (every three months during first year and every six months afterwards) as it may prevent development of advanced local recurrences.

Extra-esophageal screening does not seem to detect distant metastases in treatable stages. Shorter than one-year interval for extra-esophageal screening (especially with EUS) would probably be cost-effective and is recommended for patients with more invasive lesions (m3, sm1) who have positive distant metastasis risk.

Stomach

Early stage gastric adenocarcinoma

Literature survey

Distant recurrence

With standard indications the distant recurrence incidence was 0% in most of the studies. The estimated risk is 0.36%, which is acceptable as the mortality from surgery is higher, at 0.5% [9].

Residual tissue

Residual tissue after EMR was reported from 0% and 18%. After complete resection, the incidence of residual tissue was 0%.

Local recurrence

Local recurrence depends on resection completeness, which depends on the lesion size, EMR technique (EMR versus endoscopic submucosal dissection) and the number of resection pieces. Larger lesions resected by conventional EMR in multiple pieces have a higher frequency of incomplete or non-evaluable resections which lead to a higher rate of local recurrence. En bloc resection was complete in 81% of cases with 2% local recurrence, piecemeal resection in four pieces or more was complete in 17% of cases with 24% recurrence rate. The recurrence frequency varied from 0% to 2% for complete resection, 13% for non-evaluable lateral margin, and 37% for positive lateral margin.

Metachronous lesions
The risk of metachronous lesions after EMR may be higher than after surgery because a larger gastric surface remains. On the other hand, after Billroth-type surgery the alkaline pH will promote the formation of N-nitroso carcinogens in the stomach. The five years post-surgery cumulative prevalence rate was 2.4%.

After EMR the metachronous frequency was reported from 3.5% in 23 months to 14% in 36 months.

Metachronous lesions were usually found at the same one-third of the stomach, usually at the distal two-thirds; were differentiated; with the same macroscopic aspect and a smaller size than the initial lesion.

Most metachronous lesions were in early stages, curable by repeated EMR or surgery in the few cases with submucosal involvement or undifferentiated. Metachronous lesions were not fatal.

Micro-satellite instability (MSI) was a risk factor. Older age, presence of synchronous lesions and *Helicobacter pylori* infection were all risk factors in one study and without influence in another. Male sex was not a risk factor in two studies.

Follow-up technique and schedules
Standard endoscopy plus indigo carmine was used. Examinations were performed in the first one to two weeks to check for residual tissue. Follow-up was carried out at one, two and/or three months after EMR then at six month intervals within the first year, or not at all. After the first year, the examinations were done yearly or every six months for the first two years.

After surgery for early gastric cancer, there was a difference in patients with less than two years surveillance intervals versus patients with longer than two year intervals. Although the total number of metachronous cancers was not significantly different, the number of advanced metachronous cancers was significantly higher in the longer interval follow-up group.

Follow-up intervals used after EMR were, on average, annual. It might be thought that after EMR, shorter screening intervals could prevent development of submucosal cancers, but this may not always be true as one submucosal lesion appeared nine months after EMR [10]. On the contrary, as the differentiation rate does not depend on the size and extension of the lesion, there is no reason to believe that shorter screening intervals would prevent the development of poorly differentiated lesions as one case was found six months after a normal endoscopic examination [11].

Compliance is essential. One patient lost to follow-up was diagnosed with advanced cancer diagnosed more than 11 years after the EMR [12].

Risk groups

Patients with early gastric cancer with MSI may benefit from higher follow-up frequency.

Using closer follow-up intervals for patients with extended indications would not detect recurrent lesions in curable stages. This is sustained by the fact that in one study, four years after the EMR, a case of poorly differentiated early gastric cancer led to development of local, distant recurrence and death, which were not prevented by additional EMR, laser and a close six-month follow-up [13].

Risk modification

Although disputed, *Helicobacter pylori* infection should be looked for and eradicated.

Summary of evidence and recommendations

Early second look endoscopy is needed to look for residual tissue, even for complete en bloc resection.

The follow-up should be adapted to the resection completeness and also to the presence of risk factors for metachronous lesions. Optimal follow-up should be done at one, three and six months during the first year, then yearly.

Surgery is needed for a small proportion of early gastric cancers found through follow-up – poorly differentiated or with submucosal involvement. After surgery patient prognosis is unaffected and there is a 99% specific survival rate.

Extra-esophageal surveillance with EUS may be recommended, in a similar manner to the post-EMR follow-up for early esophageal cancers.

Ampulla and duodenum

Apart from adenomas and adenocarcinomas, other histological types of ampullary tumors are rare, their treatment by EMR is performed in a case-by-case manner and their post-EMR surveillance is not standardized. Because of the low negative predictive value of ampullary biopsies showing adenoma, EMR is primary diagnostic.

Duodenal non-ampullary lesions are also rare. Adenomas are the most frequent histological type and other than that, there may be hamartomas, Brunner's glands, inflammatory polyps and other rare lesions (leiomyoma, lypoma, lymphangioma, carcinoid tumor, neurofibroma).

Adenomas and adenocarcinomas may be familial adenomatous polyposis (FAP) associated or sporadic.

Literature survey

Distant recurrence
EMR with curative intent may be performed for sporadic or FAP-associated ampullary adenomas and adenocarcinomas with zero risk of lymph node metastasis (mucosal adenocarcinoma not extending beyond the sphincter of Oddi). For ampullary lesions, after EMR, if the lesion has a lymph node metastasis risk of more than zero, surgery is to be done (Whipple resection).

Residual tissue
If the risk of lymph node metastasis is zero, a systematic follow-up for residual tissue is performed at one to three months after EMR. Expected residual tissue rate is 0–26% of cases of EMR for ampullary lesions. If residual tissue is found, EMR is repeated until complete resection.

Local recurrence
Local recurrence rate varies from 4% for sporadic to 23% for FAP-related ampullary lesions [14]. For sporadic duodenal adenomas, local recurrences may be detected in 25% of cases, all treatable by repeated EMR.

Follow-up technique and schedules
In patients with FAP, guidelines have been published for endoscopic surveillance after colectomy [15]. This should be done every two to three years at the level of duodenum and proximal jejunum with an axial and lateral view endoscope plus chromoscopy with indigo carmine. Anomalies are graded according to Spiegelman stage [16]. In stage IV surgical resection should be discussed. In cases of duodenal or ampullary adenomas more than 10 mm or high-grade dysplasia EMR may be considered.

After EMR for sporadic duodenal adenomas different policies have been proposed: either at 1, 6 and 12 months during the first year then annually for at least 5–10 years, or every six months during the first two years and after that only when clinically indicated.

Risk modification
APC application after EMR for ampullary lesions non-significantly lowers the recurrence risk [14].

Summary of evidence and recommendations

For FAP-related duodenal or ampullary adenomas and adenocarcinomas with zero risk of distant metastasis, after complete resection follow-up is to be done yearly, at closer intervals than recommended before EMR. For sporadic ampullary adenomas, in the absence of comparative data, our opinion is that after six months surveillance during the first year, a consecutive annual surveillance may be a more safe approach.

When patients are poor candidates for surgery, EMR has a palliative intent and a palliative stent placement may be proposed, with control examinations afterward only when clinically indicated.

Colon and rectum

Benign colorectal lesions consist mainly of adenomas and hyperplastic polyps, while malignant lesions are mainly adenocarcinomas.

Literature survey

Risk groups
For adenomas, high-magnification endoscopy might predict resection completeness after EMR, with sensitivity of 80% and specificity of 97% [17].

Risk modification
Also, for adenomas, APC of the resection margins after apparent complete resection decreases the risk of local recurrence.

Celecoxib reduces metachronous recurrence of colorectal adenomas in the three years after their resection, but its use increases the risk of cardiovascular events. Moreover in a decision analysis, surveillance colonoscopy was more cost-effective than celecoxib.

Summary of evidence and recommendations

Guidelines regarding post-polypectomy surveillance [18] are also applicable post-EMR. An initial one- to three-month colonoscopy to check for residual tissue is recommended. Patients are stratified according to their risk for metachronous advanced adenomas, depending on histology, the number of adenomas, size and resection type. After complete resection, surveillance colonoscopy is to be done:

- 10 years after EMR of hyperplastic polyps
- Five to ten years after EMR in the case of one to two small tubular adenomas with low-grade dysplasia
- Three years after EMR for 3–10 adenomas or size larger than 10 mm, or villous, or with high-grade dysplasia (provided that the resection was en bloc)
- Less than three years for more than 10 adenomas (screening for familial polyposis syndromes is also necessary in this case)
- Sessile adenomas removed piecemeal at 1, 3 and 5 years.

In polyposis syndromes, EMR indication is to be discussed and if performed, surveillance is to be done according to the specific disease guideline, but essentially more frequently than for sporadic lesions [19].

Follow-up colonoscopy should be performed more frequently after EMR for lateral spreading tumors. Recurrence rate in these lesions was 17% in two years, eight of ten recurrences were retreated by EMR. Colonoscopy at three and six months during the first year is recommended and then after one, three and five years (similar to large sessile adenomas). APC at the resection margins may reduce the risk of local recurrence.

Guidelines for post-cancer resection surveillance [20] are also valid for post-EMR. An initial one- to three-month colonoscopy to check for residual tissue is needed. After complete local resection, colonoscopy surveillance is performed at 1, 3, and 5 years.

For rectal lesions more frequent examinations may be performed every three to six months during the first two to three years. EUS may be used for lymph node metastasis surveillance.

Chromoendoscopy and magnification endoscopy are not essential to screening and surveillance.

Subepithelial lesions

Literature survey

EMR of subepithelial lesions is mainly performed with a diagnostic purpose, as an alternative to the classical 'surveillance or surgery.' It can provide a histological specimen for diagnosis, significantly more frequent than with biopsy or fine needle aspiration. Noninvasive imaging techniques such as endoscopic ultrasound are essential in the pre-EMR staging, but alone cannot establish diagnosis on the basis of the image characteristics.

In the series published in the literature, the authors followed up the patients early after EMR to verify healing, then every six months during the first year and yearly afterwards or from the start at every two or three months. No recurrences were detected for benign lesions.

Malignant lesions or with malignant potential such as gastrointestinal stromal tumors (GIST), carcinoid or lymphomas are managed according to their etiology.

The malignant potential of GIST depends on its mitotic index which cannot be appreciated on biopsy fragments, but only on resected specimens. EMR is purely diagnostic in GIST lesions (it provides specimen for diagnostic and mitotic index calculation), even in R0 resection or in low-grade mitotic index. Surgery is indicated in every GIST case.

For carcinoid lesions, there have been case reports of lesions treated by EMR in various locations of the digestive tract. Adequate assessment according to published guidelines is mandatory [21]. Series of small gastric and rectal carcinoid tumors resected by EMR have been published. There have been no reports of recurrence after EMR for rectal carcinoid in a follow-up of three years. Type-1 gastric carcinoids which are smaller than 10 mm may be treated by EMR.

Summary of evidence and recommendations

Benign lesions (lipoma, fibroma, leiomyoma, etc.) do not need follow-up.

For GIST lesions, as EMR is purely diagnostic, there is no post-EMR follow-up policy. Follow-up after surgery includes CT scan every six months for five years.

Although there have been no recurrences after EMR for rectal carcinoids, intensive follow-up – yearly chest X-ray, abdominal CT scan, colonoscopy and EUS – is recommended, due to the unpredictable nature of these lesions.

After EMR for gastric carcinoids, follow-up after EMR is warranted, but there is no established schedule. A six month follow-up interval is recommended.

References

1 Seewald S, Akaraviputh T, Seitz U et al. Circumferential EMR and complete removal of Barrett's epithelium: a new approach to management of Barrett's esophagus containing high-grade intraepithelial neoplasia and intramucosal carcinoma. Gastrointest Endosc 2003; 57: 854–9.
2 Giovannini M, Bories E, Presenti C et al. Circumferential endoscopic mucosal resection in Barrett's esophagus with high-grade intraepithelial neoplasia or mucosal cancer. Preliminary results in 21 patients. Endoscopy 2004; 36: 782–7.
3 Shimizu Y, Tsukagoshi M et al. Metachronous squamous cell carcinoma of the esophagus arising after endoscopic mucosal resection. Gastrointest Endosc 2001; 54: 190–94.

4 Shimizu Y, Tsukagoshi H, Fujita M *et al.* Long-term outcome after endoscopic mucosal resection in patients with esophageal squamous cell carcinoma invading the muscularis mucosae or deeper. *Gastrointest Endosc* 2002; **56**: 387–90.

5 Pech O, May A, Gossner L *et al.* Curative endoscopic therapy in patients with early esophageal squamous-cell carcinoma or high-grade intraepithelial neoplasia. *Endoscopy* 2007; **39**: 30–5.

6 Esaki M, Matsumoto T, Hirakawa K *et al.* Risk factors for local recurrence of superficial esophageal cancer after treatment by endoscopic mucosal resection. *Endoscopy* 2007; **39**: 41–5.

7 Ciocirlan M, Lapalus MG, Hervieu V *et al.* Endoscopic mucosal resection for squamous premalignant and early malignant lesions of the esophagus. *Endoscopy* 2007; **39**: 24–9.

8 Katada C, Muto M, Manabe T *et al.* Local recurrence of squamous-cell carcinoma of the esophagus after EMR. *Gastrointest Endosc* 2005; **61**: 219–25.

9 Yamao T, Shirao K, Ono H *et al.* Risk factors for lymph node metastasis from intramucosal gastric carcinoma. *Cancer* 1996; **77**: 602–6.

10 Nasu J, Doi T, Endo H *et al.* Characteristics of metachronous multiple early gastric cancers after endoscopic mucosal resection. *Endoscopy* 2005; **37(10)**: 990–3.

11 Nakajima T, Oda I, Hamanaka H *et al.* Metachronous gastric cancers after endoscopic resection: how effective is annual endoscopic surveillance? *Gastric Cancer* 2006; **9**: 93–8.

12 Uedo N, Iishi H, Tatsuta M *et al.* Long-term outcomes after endoscopic mucosal resection for early gastric cancer. *Gastric Cancer* 2006; **9**: 88–92.

13 Murakami S, Tanabe S, Koizumi W *et al.* Endoscopic mucosal resection (EMR) for the management of poorly differentiated adenocarcinoma of the stomach: a patient who had recurrence and died 4 years after the EMR. *Gastric Cancer* 2003; **6**: 113–16.

14 Catalano MF, Linder JD, Chak A *et al.* Endosocpic management of adenoma of the major duodenal papilla. *Gastroinest Endosc* 2004; **59**: 225–32.

15 Saurin JC, Napoleon B, Gay G *et al.* Endoscopic management of patients with familial adenomatous polyposis (FAP) following a colectomy. *Endoscopy* 2005; **37(5)**: 499–501.

16 Spiegelman AD, Williams CB, Talbot IC *et al.* Upper gastrointestinal cancer in patients with familial adenomatous polyposis. *Lancet* 1989; **2**: 783–5.

17 Hurlstone DP, Cross SS, Brown S *et al.* A prospective evaluation of high-magnification choromoscopic colonoscopy in predicting completeness of EMR. *Gastrointest Endosc* 2004; **59**: 642–50.

18 Winawer SJ, Zauber AG, Fletcher RH *et al.* Guidelines for colonoscopy surveillance after polypectomy: a consensus update by the US multi-society task force on colorectal cancer and the American cancer society. *Gastroenterology* 2006; **130**: 1872–85.

19 Dunlop MG. Guidance on gastrointestinal surveillance for hereditary non-polyposis colorectal cancer, familial adenomatous polyposis, juvenile polyposis and Peutz-Jegers syndrome. *Gut* 2002; **51**: 21–7.

20 Rex DK, Kahi CJ, Levin B *et al.* Guidelines for colonoscopy surveillance after cancer resection: a consensus update by the American cancer society and the US multi-task force on colorectal cancer. *Gastroenterology* 2006; **130**: 1865–71.

21 Ramage JK, Davies AHG, Ardill J *et al.* Guidelines for the management of gastroenteropancreatic neuroendocrine (including carcinoid) tumors. *Gut* 2005; **54**: 1–16.

CHAPTER 12

Endoscopic Submucosal Dissection

HELMUT MESSMANN

Clinical results

Early esophageal cancer and tumors of the esophagogastric junction

Endoscopic submucosal dissection (ESD) in the esophagus and esophagogastric junction is more difficult due to the narrow lumen, and is associated with higher complication rates (e.g. perforation rate) compared to ESD in the stomach. Therefore up to now only limited data have been available in this area because many groups first start with ESD in the stomach. Nevertheless the aim for endoscopic treatment of early tumors in the esophagus and esophagogastric junction are similar: R0 resection of the tumors to avoid local recurrences. The EMR method for treatment of early esophageal cancer and tumors of the esophagogastric junction is safe but has its limitations. The mean resected specimen size is about 15–16 mm using either the cap or ligation technique [1]. Therefore for larger lesions piecemeal resection is performed, however en bloc resection is only possible in 23–57% and the local recurrence rate varies between 7.8% and 20% [2,3]. In the esophagus the indication for ESD or EMR depends on the histology of the esophageal cancer, since the risk for lymph node metastases in squamous cell cancer is different from Barrett's adenocarcinoma. The Japanese Esophagus Association decided that the indication for EMR or ESD should be restricted to tumors involving the superficial epithelial layer m1 (carcinoma in situ) or the proper mucosal layer (m2) in patients with squamous cell cancer of the esophagus [4]. In contrast, in patients with adenocarcinoma of a Barrett's esophagus all types of mucosal cancer (m1–3) and even invasion of the superficial submucosa up to 200 μm (sm1) local resection is allowed since lymph node metastases are quite rare in this situation [5].

Endoscopic Mucosal Resection. Edited by M. Conio, P. Siersema, A. Repici and T. Ponchon. © 2008 Blackwell Publishing. ISBN 978-1-4051-5885-5.

Since ESD is very popular in Japan and squamous cell cancer of the esophagus is more frequent compared to Barrett's esophagus adenocarcinoma, it is conclusive that the first series on ESD and esophageal cancer has been reported from a Japanese group who treated 102 patients with squamous cell cancer of the esophagus [6]. The median size of the resected specimen and cancer was 32 mm (range 8–76 mm) and 28 mm (range 4–64 mm), respectively. The en bloc resection rate was 95% (95 of 102) and the local recurrence rate was 0% (0 of 102) after a mean follow-up of 21 months (range 3–54 months). There were no perforations, but six cases of mediastinal emphysema (6%) were observed and treated conservatively. Seven patients required balloon dilation due to stenosis. The mucosa defect was 80% of the circumference in these cases.

Fujishiro et al. recently reported on 43 patients with 58 esophageal squamous cell neoplasms [7]. The rate of en bloc resection was 100% (58/58) and the en bloc resection with tumor-free lateral/basal margins (R0 resection) was 78% (45/58). There was no evidence of significant bleeding, but perforation occurred in four cases (6.9%). In all cases this complication was managed conservatively after endoscopic closure of the perforation. In nine cases (16%) ESD was associated with esophageal stricture requiring balloon dilatation. Of 40 lesions occurring in 31 patients fullfilling the criteria of node negative tumors (mean follow-up of 17 months) one lesion resected by en bloc resection with non-evaluable tumor-free lateral margins (Rx [lateral] resection) recurred locally six months after ESD, which was treated successfully by a second ESD.

Up to now no larger series on ESD and treatment of Barrett's adenocarcinoma have been available. Kakushima et al. recently published their experience on ESD in tumors of the esophagogastric junction [8]. Thirty lesions with an average diameter of 22.4 mm were resected. The size of the specimens were on average 40.6 mm in diameter and en bloc resection (R0) was possible in 97% (29/30). Perforation occurred in one case and was managed conservatively by rotable clips and antibiotics for three days. Local recurrence was not observed during follow-up (mean 16.6 months, range 6–31 months).

Early gastric cancer

Gastrectomy with lymph node dissection has provided an excellent therapeutic outcome for patients with early gastric cancer, with a five-year survival rate of 96%. The prevalence of lymph node metastases associated with intramucosal- and submucosal-invading gastric cancer was reported as approximately 1–3% and 11–20%, respectively [9]. Because of its risks and the negative effect on the quality of life that gastrectomy has, endoscopic treatment of early gastric cancer has meanwhile an accepted standard in Japan and is becoming more attractive in the Western world as well. Similar to

Table 12.1 Early gastric cancer with no risk of lymph node metastases [12].

	Incidence (no. with metastases/total number)	95% confidence interval
Intramucosal G1/G2; LO,VO; ulcer +/−; <3 cm	0/1230; 0%	0–0.3
Intramucosal G1/G2; LO,VO; ulcer-; irrespective of tumor size	0/929; 0%	0–0.4
Intramucosal ≥G3; LO,VO; ulcer-; <3 cm	0/256; 0%	0–2.6
Submucosal (Sm1) G1/G2; LO,VO; ulcer-; <3 cm	0/145; 0%	0–2.5

esophageal cancer the risk of positive lymph nodes depends on the penetration depth of the tumor. According to the *Gastric Cancer Treatment Guidelines* (GL) published by the Japanese Gastric Cancer Association in 2001, the indications for EMR of EGC are restricted to a non-ulcerated, differentiated-type mucosal carcinoma measuring ≤ 2cm [10]. Submucosal invasion, ulceration, and undifferentiated type are important risk factors for lymph node metastasis as shown in large surgical studies [11]. Using ESD as a novel approach to resect larger specimens in one piece the size of the tumor is no longer limited to 2 cm in diameter. Furthermore Gotoda analysed more than 5000 patients who underwent gastrectomy with R2-level lymph node dissection and found further criteria to extend the indication for endoscopic treatment of gastric cancer [12]. Table 12.1 shows different criteria and the risk for lymph node metastases.

Meanwhile ESD is performed in many centers in Japan since it offers the advantage of R0- en bloc resection and reduces the risk for recurrences compared to EMR.

The technique and especially the equipment are still changing, which demonstrates that ESD in its present form can still be improved. Meanwhile quite a lot of knifes (insulated-tip knife, flex-knife, triangle-knife, and hook-knife) have been developed and many centers prefer their 'own knife' for ESD. The first large series came from the National Cancer Center Hospital, where the IT-knife was developed. In the first series on 41 patients complete resection of the tumors was dependent on the tumor size: one-piece resection rates were 82% (14/17) for lesions ≤10 mm, 75% (12/16) for those between 11 and 20 mm and 14% (1/7) for those of ≥20 mm [13]. In their following series they could improve their complete en bloc resection rates for lesions ≥20 mm to 76% (22/29), demonstrating that ESD needs a special learning curve [14]. Rösch *et al.*

also had initially disappointing results with complete resection rates of only 25% in a series of 24 mucosa lesions [15]. Recent data from Ono using the IT knife demonstrated a complete resection in one piece in 96% (471/488) [16]. Watanabe compared the ESD with historical data of conventional EMR. The complete en bloc resection rates were significantly higher in the ESD group compared to the EMR group, however the procedure was more time consuming for lesions larger than 10 mm [17].

The most important factor for successful en bloc resection is the experience of the endoscopist. It is not associated with tumor location/site, tumor size, specimen size, or ulceration within the tumor [18]. In this study, in 9% en bloc resection by ESD failed. The multivariate analysis showed that the second-half period of the procedure was responsible for the success. Finally in cases with recurrent early gastric cancer after prior EMR it was possible to treat those patients more effectively with ESD than with EMR. Among 46 patients who underwent ESD, 41 (89.1%) en bloc resections were achieved but in none of the 18 cases who were retreated by conventional EMR. One specimen out of 41 (2.4%) cases treated by ESD was not evaluable, compared to 10 lesions of 23 piecemeal resections ($p < 0.0001$) [19].

The two major complications of ESD are bleeding and perforation. Bleeding is the most common complication, occurring in up to 8% of patients undergoing standard EMR and in up to 7% of patients undergoing ESD [20]. During ESD, immediate minor bleeding is not uncommon but can be successfully treated by grasping and coagulation of the bleeding vessels using hot biopsy forceps. Delayed bleeding is commonly found after ESD, but is strongly dependent on the location and size of the tumor [21]. Perforation during EMR is rare but occurs more often during ESD (4%), but in most cases endoscopic clipping of the defect is possible.

Colorectal neoplasia

The experience with ESD in the colorectum is limited. Yamamoto reported on a case of a large villous tumor of the sigmoid which was treated by ESD using a hyaluronic acid and a small-caliber-tip transparent hood. The resected specimen was an intra-mucosal well-differentiated adenocarcinoma with a 70×55 mm diameter [22] and another case of a 40-mm flat-elevated tumor in the rectum [23]. Recently, Fujishiro reported on a larger series of rectal epithelial neoplasia treated by ESD: 35 consecutive patients were treated with ESD. The rates of en bloc resection and en bloc plus R0 resection were 88.6% (31 of 35) and 62.9% (22 of 35), respectively. No major bleeding requiring blood transfusion occurred, but two patients suffered from perforation (5.7%), and were managed conservatively. In three patients with sm2 or deeper infiltration, surgery was performed. The remaining 32 patients were free of recurrence during a mean follow-up of 36 months (range 12–60 months) [24].

Submucosal tumors

ESD has the potential to enucleate submucosal tumors in a R0 situation. While Rösch et al. [15] reported disappointing data on 14 patients with submucosal tumors and 36% R0 resection, Park et al. [25] could enucleate 14 of 15 tumors completely. The median procedure time in the series from Park was 35 min (8–160 min) and the median size 2×1.7 cm. The largest lesion located in the esophagus measured 6×3 cm. Histopathologic diagnosis included leiomyoma (9), GIST (4), stromal tumor of unknown malignant potential (1), and glomus tumor (1). One perforation occurred in a patient with a 2.5 cm tumor in the anterior wall of the stomach but could be managed by clip application. En bloc endoscopic enucleation of submucosal tumors by using an insulated-tip electrosurgical knife appears to be safer, easier, and less time consuming compared with previously described methods.

Conclusion

ESD is a novel technique that allows en bloc resection of large mucosal/submucosal tumors in the stomach, esophagus, and colon. The advantage of this technique is the low recurrence rate after endoscopic treatment, however there are also some disadvantages. The procedure is only safe in experienced hands since the complication rate of bleeding and especially perforation is higher compared to conventional EMR. Therefore the procedure needs a relative long learning curve and is time consuming. Improvement of the technical equipment will overcome the disadvantages in the near future.

References

1 May A, Gossner L, Behrens A et al. A prospective randomized trial of two different endoscopic resection techniques for early stage cancer of the esophagus. *Gastrointest Endosc* 2003; 58: 167–75.
2 Takeo Y, Yoshida T, Shigemitu T, Yanai H, Hayashi N, Okita K. Endoscopic mucosal resection for early esophageal cancer and esophageal dysplasia. *Hepatogastroenterology* 2001; 48: 453–7.
3 Nomura T, Boku N, Ohtsu A, Muto M, Matsumoto S, Tajiri H, Yoshida S. Recurrence after endoscopic mucosal resection for superficial esophageal cancer. *Endoscopy* 2000; 32: 277–80.
4 Japanese Society for Esophageal Disease. *Guidelines for Clinical and Pathological Studies on Carcinoma of the Esophagus* [in Japanese] 9th edn. Kanehara Shuppan, Tokyo, 1999.
5 Endoscopic classification review group. Update on the Paris classification of superficial neoplastic lesions in the digestive tract. *Endoscopy* 2005; 37: 570–8.
6 Oyama T, Tomori A, Hotta K et al. Endoscopic submucosal dissection of early esophageal cancer. *Clin Gastroenterol Hepatol* 2005; 3(7Suppl 1): S67–70.

7 Fujishiro M, Yahagi N, Kakushima N *et al*. Endoscopic submucosal dissection of esophageal squamous cell neoplasms. *Clin Gastroenterol Hepatol* 2006; **4**: 688–94.

8 Kakushima N, Yahagi N, Fujishiro M, Kodashima S, Nakamura M, Omata M. Efficacy and safety of endoscopic submucosal dissection for tumors of the esophagogastric junction. *Endoscopy* 2006; **38**: 170–4.

9 Adachi Y, Shiraishi N, Kitano S. Modern treatment of early gastric cancer: review of the Japanese experience. *Dig Surg* 2002; **19**: 333–9.

10 Japanese Gastric Cancer Association. *Guidelines for the Treatment of Gastric Cancer*. Kanehara & Co., Tokyo, 2001.

11 Yamao T, Shirao K, Ono H *et al*. Risk factors for lymph node metastasis from intramucosal gastric carcinoma. *Cancer* 1996; **77**: 602–6.

12 Gotoda T, Yanagisawa A, Sasako M *et al*. Incidence of lymph node metastasis from early gastric cancer: estimation with a large number of cases at two large centers. *Gastric Cancer* 2000; **3**: 219–25.

13 Ohkuwa M, Hosokawa K, Boku N, Ohtu A, Tajiri H, Yoshida S. New endoscopic treatment for intramucosal gastric tumors using an insulated-tip diathermic knife. *Endoscopy* 2001; **33**: 221–6.

14 Miyamoto S, Muto M, Hamamoto Y *et al*. A new technique for endoscopic mucosal resection with an insulated-tip electrosurgical knife improves the completeness of resection of intramucosal gastric neoplasms. *Gastrointest Endosc* 2002; **55**: 576–81.

15 Rösch T, Sarbia M, Schumacher B, Deinert K, Frimberger E, Toermer T, Stolte M, Neuhaus H. Attempted endoscopic en bloc resection of mucosal and submucosal tumors using insulated-tip knives: a pilot series. *Endoscopy* 2004; **36**: 788–801.

16 Ono H. Endoscopic submucosal dissection for early gastric cancer. *Chin J Dig Dis* 2005; **6**: 119–21.

17 Watanabe K, Ogata S, Kawazoe S *et al*. Clinical outcomes of EMR for gastric tumors: historical pilot evaluation between endoscopic submucosal dissection and conventional mucosal resection. *Gastrointest Endosc* 2006; **63**: 776–82.

18 Abe N, Yamaguchi Y, Takeuchi H *et al*. Key factors for successful en bloc endoscopic submucosal dissection of early stage gastric cancer using an insulation-tipped diathermic knife. *Hepatogastroenterology* 2006; **53**: 639–42.

19 Yokoi C, Gotoda T, Hamanaka H, Oda I. Endoscopic submucosal dissection allows curative resection of locally recurrent early gastric cancer after prior endoscopic mucosal resection. *Gastrointest Endosc* 2006; **64**: 212–18.

20 Oda I, Gotoda T, Hamanaka H. Endoscopic submucosal dissection for early gastric cancer: technical feasibility, operation time and complications from a large consecutive series. *Dig Endosc* 2005; **17**: 54–58.

21 Shiba M, Higuchi K, Kadouchi K *et al*. Risk factors for bleeding after endoscopic mucosal resection. *World J Gastroenterol* 2005; **14**: 7335–9.

22 Yamamoto H, Kawata H, Sunada K *et al*. Successful en-bloc resection of large superficial tumors in the stomach and colon using sodium hyaluronate and small-caliber-tip transparent hood. *Endoscopy* 2003; **35**: 690–4.

23 Yamamoto H, Koiwai H, Yube T *et al*. A successful single-step endoscopic resection of a 40 millimeter flat-elevated tumor in the rectum: endoscopic mucosal resection using sodium hyaluronate. *Gastrointest Endosc* 1999; **50**: 701–4.

24 Fujishiro M, Yahagi N, Nakamura M *et al*. Endoscopic submucosal dissection for rectal epithelial neoplasia. *Endoscopy* 2006; **38**: 493–7.

25 Park YS, Park SW, Kim TI *et al*. Endoscopic enucleation of upper-GI submucosal tumors by using an insulated-tip electrosurgical knife. *Gastrointest Endosc* 2004; **59**: 409–15.

CHAPTER 13

EMR and ESD for Early Gastrointestinal Cancers

SERGIO CODA, ICHIRO ODA, TAKUJI GOTODA, AND YUTAKA SAITO

Introduction

Endoscopic resection (ER) has been accepted as a less invasive local resection in early cancers of the gastrointestinal tract, with a negligible risk of lymph node metastasis [1–3]. This allows less invasive treatments and therefore improves the quality of life of the patients when compared with surgery. The method of ER varies from polypectomy and conventional endoscopic mucosal resection (EMR) to endoscopic submucosal dissection (ESD) [4–14]. EMR procedures include inject and cut, strip biopsy, EMR with a cap-fitted panendoscope (EMR-C), endoscopic aspiration mucosectomy (EAM), and EMR with a ligating device (EMRL). ESD is a new method of ER developed for achieving one-piece resection, especially in the stomach.

In this chapter, we describe ER for early cancers of the gastrointestinal tract especially focusing on technical points of ESD for early gastric cancer (EGC).

Stomach

EMR and ESD are established alternative treatments to surgery for EGC in Japan [15]. The general criteria for EMR in EGC proposed by the Japanese Gastric Cancer Association includes: (1) differentiated adenocarcinoma; (2) intramucosal cancer; (3) lesion less than 20 mm in size; and (4) without ulcer finding [16]. Lesions that meet all of the above criteria have a negligible risk of lymph node metastasis and have a reasonable tumor size that will allow one-piece resection by conventional EMR. Recently, based on the risk of lymph node metastasis in

Endoscopic Mucosal Resection. Edited by M. Conio, P. Siersema, A. Repici and T. Ponchon. © 2008 Blackwell Publishing. ISBN 978-1-4051-5885-5.

Table 13.1 Expanded histological criteria for curative endoscopic resection.

1. Differentiated adenocarcinoma

    and

2. No lymphatic or venous invasion

    and

3. Intramucosal cancer regardless of tumor size without ulcer finding

    or

    Intramucosal cancer ≤30 mm in size with ulcer finding

    or

    Minute submucosal cancer (sm1) ≤30 mm in size

    and

4. Tumor-free margin

EGC obtained from a large number of surgical cases, expanded histological criteria for ER in EGC have been reported (Table 13.1) [17]. These include lesions of more than 20 mm in size and ulcerative lesions which were originally resected by surgery. By expanding the criteria for EMR as suggested above, the need for gastrectomy in EGC can be reduced, as these patients could be treated by EMR. However, it is difficult to resect large and ulcerative lesions by conventional EMR techniques so a new technique of endoscopic submucosal dissection (ESD) has been developed [9–15].

The primary aim of the ESD technique is to obtain one-piece resection during ER. Despite requiring significant additional technical skill and a longer procedure time [18,19], these ESD techniques are rapidly gaining popularity in Japan, primarily because of the ability to remove large EGC lesions en bloc. ESD utilizes a direct dissection of the submucosa with a modified needle knife. ESD with an insulation-tipped (IT) diathermic knife (see Chapter 7, Fig. 7.3(a)), developed at the National Cancer Center Hospital, was the first of these techniques [9–11,20]. The concept of ESD with an IT knife was initially proposed and modified to make ERHSE, usually performed by a surgeon, easier and safer to perform by an endoscopist. Other endoscopic devices for the ESD procedure, a hook-knife (Chapter 7, Fig. 7.3(b)) [13], a flex-knife (Fig. 7.3(c)) [14], and a needle knife in a small cap technique [12], have also been described. The processes of ESD differ depending on endoscopic devices such as IT knife, hook-knife, flex knife, and so on.

We describe in particular the established ESD technique with IT knife for en bloc resection and comment on the set-up of the high-frequency electric surgical unit (Table 13.2). The process of ESD consists of three steps: (1) identification of the lesion margin and marking with the needle knife (Fig. 13.1(a)); (2) the mucosa is then lifted up by submucosal fluid injection followed by a circumferential incision (Fig. 13.1(b)); and (3) Submucosal dissection under the lesion is performed with the IT knife (Fig. 13.1(c)–(f)).

Table 13.2 Set-up of high-frequency electric surgical unit of ESD with IT knife for early gastric cancer.

Procedure	Device	Mode	Output
(a) ICC200; ERBE Corp., Tubingen, Germany			
Marking	Needle knife	Forced coag	20 W
Precutting	Needle knife	ENDO CUT	Effect 3, 80 W
Mucosal incision	IT knife	ENDO CUT	Effect 3, 80 W
	Needle knife		
Submucosal dissection	IT knife	ENDO CUT	Effect 3, 80 W
		Forced coag	50W
	Needle knife	ENDO CUT	Effect 3, 80 W
		Forced coag	50 W
Endoscopic hemostasis	IT knife	Forced coag	50 W
	Needle knife		
	Hot biopsy Coagrasper	Soft coag	80 W
(b) VIO300D; ERBE Corp., Tubingen, Germany			
Marking	Needle knife	Swift coag	Effect 2, 50 W
Precutting	Needle knife	ENDO CUT I	Effect 2, CUT duration 3, CUT interval 1
Mucosal incision	IT knife	ENDO CUT I or Q	Effect 2, CUT duration 3, CUT interval 1
		DRY CUT	Effect 4, 50 W
	Needle knife	ENDO CUT I	Effect 2, CUT duration 3, CUT interval 1
Submucosal dissection	IT knife	DRY CUT	Effect 4, 50 W
		ENDO CUTI or Q	Effect 2, CUT duration 3, CUT interval 1
		DRY CUT	Effect 4, 50 W
		Swift coag	Effect 5, 50 W
	Needle knife	ENDO CUT I	Effect 2, CUT duration 3, CUT interval 1
		DRY CUT	Effect 4, 50 W
		Swift coag	Effect 5, 50 W
Endoscopic hemostasis	IT knife	Swift coag	Effect 5, 50 W
	Needle knife		
	Hot biopsy Coagrasper	Soft coag	Effect 5, 80 W

Needle knife (KD-1L-1; Olympus Medical Systems Corp., Tokyo, Japan); IT knife (KD-610L; Olympus Medical Systems Corp., Tokyo, Japan); Hot biopsy forceps (Radial Jaw; Boston Scientific Corp., Natick, Mass.); Coagrasper (FD-410LR; Olympus Medical Systems Corp., Tokyo, Japan).

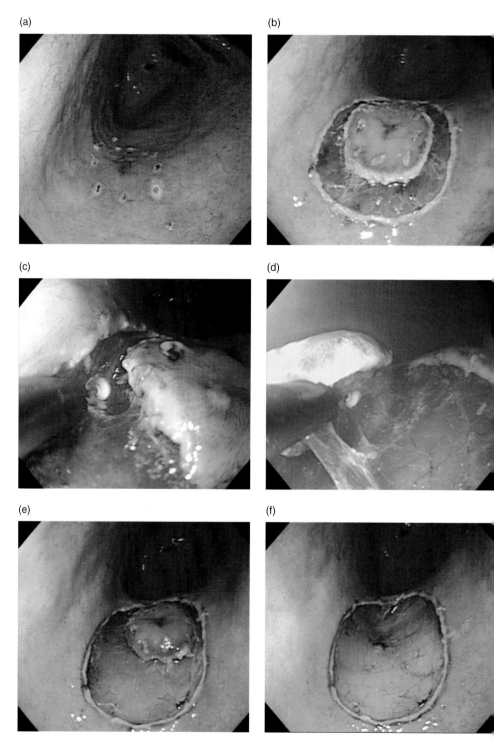

Fig. 13.1 Process of ESD: (a) Marking of the periphery of the lesion; (b) Submucosal fluid injection and mucosal incision; (c)–(e) Submucosal dissection; (f) Mucosal defect of resected site.

1   Marking of the periphery of the lesion is begun by using a standard needle knife with 50W of forced coagulation mode (ICC200; ERBE Corp., Tubingen, Germany).

2   After injection of normal saline mixed with epinephrine and indigo carmine to raise the submucosal layer, a small initial incision is made by a standard needle knife with 80W of endocut mode with effect 3 (ICC200; ERBE Corp., Tubingen, Germany) for insertion of the tip of the IT knife into the submucosal layer. We usually use dilute 1 mg of epinephrine and 1–4 ml of 0.4% indigo carmine solution with 200 ml of normal saline. The concentration of epinephrine for ESD is lower than that for EMR, because we sometimes need a lot of injection solution during ESD. The use of fluid solution mixed with indigo carmine for submucosal injection is effective to distinguish the white muscularis propria from the blue submucosal layer during following submucosal dissection (Fig. 13.1(d)). The concentration of indigo carmine solution depends on operator preference. Then circumferential mucosal cutting at the periphery of the marking dots is performed by an IT knife with 80W of endocut mode with effect 3 (ICC200; ERBE Corp., Tubingen, Germany).

3   After completion of the circumferential cutting, normal saline is injected again submucosally. With the same IT knife, the submucosal layer under the lesion is directly dissected using a lateral movement. Complete endoscopic submucosal dissection can achieve a large one-piece resection without size limitation. Finally, the resected specimen is retrieved with grasping forceps.

More tips

1   Marking of the periphery of the lesion with a stronger press and too much coagulation by the needle knife may sometimes cause a minor perforation. Marking with other devices such as argon plasma coagulation (APC), hook knife, or flex knife is also useful to prevent a minor perforation.

2   A first incision by needle knife should be located on the far point on the TV monitor, because following mucosal incision using an IT knife is performed from the far side to near side. For example, the first incision should be located on a distal side of the lesion when located on the gastric antrum (Fig. 13.2(a)). On the other hand it should be on a proximal side of the lesion when located on the gastric body, because we need a retroflex view (Fig. 13.2(b)). A superficial initial incision should not be done, because it makes it difficult following mucosal incision by IT knife.

3   The IT knife should be placed from a tangential position not from a vertical position to get an adequate depth of mucosal incision (Fig. 13.3).

(a)

(b)

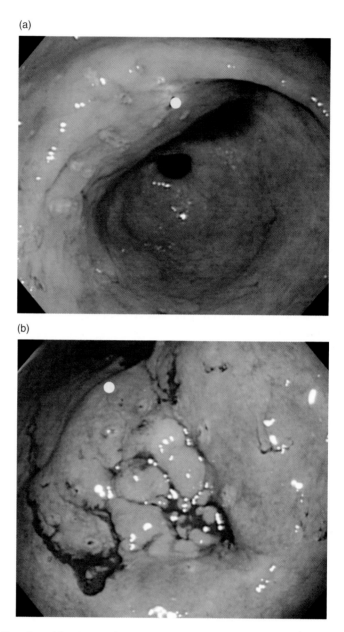

Fig. 13.2 Location of first incision by needle knife: (a) Distal side of the lesion when it is located on the gastric antrum; (b) proximal side of the lesion when it is located on the gastric body.

(b)

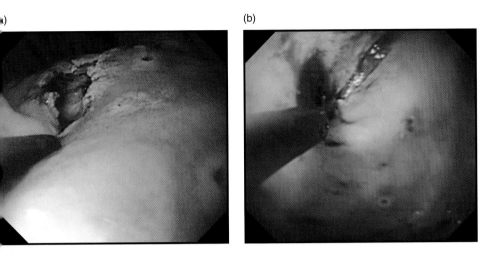

ig. 13.3   Position of IT knife: (a) Proper example (placed from tangential position); (b) improper example placed from vertical position).

4   Because submucosal dissection using an IT knife is performed from the far side to the near side on the TV monitor, it is easy to do it lengthwise but difficult to do it widthwise. Therefore we would start with submucosal dissection lengthwise from the far side, make a hole at the near side, and then continue to dissect widthwise, hanging the IT knife on the hole (Fig. 13.1(c),(d)). The perforation induced by ESD usually occurs during the process of submucosal dissection and not during circumferential incision. The potential mechanisms of perforation induced by ESD are submucosal dissection with less space in the submucosal layer and misunderstanding of the gastric wall curve. The fluid solution mixed with indigo carmine for submucosal injection can be injected into the submucosa at any time to raise and confirm the submucosal layer. It is important to cut tangentially to the submucosal layer to avoid perforation. The use of transparent attachment of the scope is useful to recognize the gastric wall curve. It is also useful to get counter-traction for easier dissection.

Esophagus

Squamous cell carcinoma (SCC) of the esophagus that is confined to m1 and m2 is a definite indication for ER. Nodal metastases were found in 0% of patients with m1 and m2 SCC of the esophagus, 8% with m3, and 30% with sm1 tumors [21]. Following EMR in patients with superficial SCC, the five-year survival rate is up to 95% [22,23]. EMR in 25 patients with superficial m1 SCC showed no recurrence after a mean follow-up of two years [24]. It has been reported that patients with m3 areas infiltrating the muscularis mucosa (MM) showed lymph node or distal metastasis. These patients should be treated with curative surgery [25]. Few reports have analyzed the outcome of EMR in patients with invasive cancer. Shimizu *et al.* compared 26 patients with SCC invading the MM or the submucosa, treated by EMR, with 44 comparable patients undergoing surgery. Survival was similar in the two groups: 77% vs. 84% [26]. Esophageal stenosis developed after endoscopic mucosal resection in 13 lesions (6.0%). During the follow-up period (median 26 months), no patient died of esophageal cancer. Recently, an expansion of the indications for EMR in patients with superficial esophageal carcinoma m3 or sm1 has been proposed in Japan [27]. Multiple synchronous lesions have been reported in 26–31% of patients with SCC [28]. We should also be careful with metachronous lesions. The application of ESD for esophageal SCC has been reported with promising results [29].

Colorectum

EMR and ESD are being successfully used for early-stage colon cancers, flat adenomas, large superficial colorectal tumors, and rectal carcinoids [30,31]. Lymph node metastasis in T1 colorectal carcinoma occurs only after infiltration of the submucosa and is correlated to the depth of submucosal penetration by the tumor. This supports the therapeutic effectiveness of endoscopic removal of polyps and flat lesions when confined to the mucosa, regardless of their size [32]. Some authors prefer snare excision without cap. Of 57 patients with sessile polyps (SP) and early cancers of 10–50 mm, complications occurred in 2 patients [33]. Published studies show a recurrence rate following EMR ranging from 0% to 40% [34,35]. Combined APC reduced the recurrence rate by 50% [36,37]. In another report, APC did not reduce the recurrence rate compared to polypectomy alone [38]. EMR was performed for 139 SP in 136 patients by snare polypectomy, with or without cap. Median lesion diameter was 20 mm in the right colon and 30 mm in the remaining bowel. Bleeding occurred in 11%. Invasive carcinoma was found in 17 SP, and surgery was performed in 10 of these. After a median 12 months, local recurrence was detected in 22% of polyps with no invasive cancer, and in none of the patients with alonocarcinoma who did not undergo surgery [39]. Of EMR in 24 patients with 30 large colorectal polyps (median size 20 mm), 22 lesions were resected en bloc while 8 were resected piecemeal. Histologically the lesions were predominantly adenomatous polyps. An incidental focus of ADC was found in seven lesions. Histologically complete excision was achieved in 10 lesions. Bleeding occurred during two EMRs. There was no case of bowel perforation. Median follow-up period was 21 months. None of the patients diagnosed with ADC showed any evidence of recurrence [40].

Colorectal laterally spreading tumors (LSTs), classified in granular and non-granular type, are defined as lesions larger than 10 mm in diameter, with a low vertical axis, extending along the luminal wall. They are best removed by ESD as they sometimes invade deeply into the submucosal layer. For en bloc resection of flat lesions >20 mm, conventional EMR is inadequate because incomplete removal and local recurrence are frequently observed. When analyzing the endoscopic features of 257 LSTs in order to assess which features correlated with the depth of invasion, unevenness of nodules, presence of large nodules, size, histological type, and presence of depression in the tumor were significantly associated with depth of invasion. When LSTs showed even nodules without depression, or uneven nodules without depression and less than 3 mm in diameter, the risk of massive submucosal invasion was 0% (0/121) and 3.7% (3/82) respectively. When LSTs meet the above endoscopic criteria, ESD should be the first-line treatment because of the low risk of submucosal invasion [41]. In a recent study, LSTs non-granular type (LST-NG) showed a higher frequency of submucosal invasion than granular (LST-G) (14% versus 7%). Presence of a large nodule in LST-G type was associated with higher submucosal invasion while pit pattern (invasive), sclerous wall change, and larger size were significantly associated with higher sm invasion in LST-NG type. In LST-G type with sm invasion, sm penetration occurred under the largest nodules and depressed areas. Therefore, for LST-G type, endoscopic piecemeal resection with the area including the large nodule resected first is advisable. In contrast, LST-NG type should be removed by ESD en bloc because of the higher potential of sm invasion compared with LST-G type [31,42]. We need some improvements for ESD in the colorectum because of its technical difficulty and the risk of perforation. As an injection solution a mixed solution with glycerol and sodium hyaluronate acid should be used to keep better lifting. The newly developed B-knife results in a safer ESD, because the electric current is localized to the needle tip [31]. CO_2 insufflation instead of air insufflation is used for safer ESD and for reducing patient discomfort [43]. In a recent prospective study in Italy, the IT knife was used for EMR of large colorectal polyps (>3 cm) unsuitable for standard polypectomy [44]. The results of this pilot study showed that the likelihood of complete en bloc resection of mucosal lesions is improved by this new approach compared with previous studies on colonic EMR, even for lesions located in difficult positions or larger than 30 mm. En bloc resection was achieved in 55.1% of the lesions and in the other cases piecemeal resection was used. Thirteen patients had low-grade dysplasia, fifteen had high-grade dysplasia, and one had a tumor invading the submucosa and was admitted to surgery. Complications occurred in four patients (13.7%), all managed conservatively. Local recurrence was detected in five patients (17.8%) and was treated by APC and snare polypectomy. No further recurrence was observed over the median follow-up period of 15.7 months.

Conclusion

For all gastrointestinal cancers, prognosis correlates with stage of the disease at diagnosis. With the discovery of these early lesions, EMR and ESD could be used with increasing frequency, avoiding surgery with its relatively high mortality and morbidity. In conclusion, the EMR and ESD techniques, if performed with the right indications and with expertise, should be considered as an elective treatment modality for early gastrointestinal cancers.

References

1 Rembacken BJ, Gotoda T, Fujii T, Axon AT. Endoscopic mucosal resection. *Endoscopy* 2001; **33**: 709–18.

2 Soetikno RM, Gotoda T, Nakanishi Y, Soehendra N. Endoscopic mucosal resection. *Gastrointest Endosc* 2003; **57**: 567–79.

3 Conio M, Ponchon T, Blanchi S, Filiberti R. Endoscopic mucosal resection. *Am J Gastroenterol* 2006; **101**: 653–63.

4 Deyhle P, Largiader F, Jenny S, Fumagalli I. A method for endoscopic electroresection of sessile colonic polyps. *Endoscopy* 1973; **5**: 38–40.

5 Tada M, Murakami A, Karita M, Yanai H, Okita K. Endoscopic resection of early gastric cancer. *Endoscopy* 1993; **25**: 445–51.

6 Inoue H, Takeshita K, Hori H, Muraoka Y, Yoneshima H, Endo M. Endoscopic mucosal resection with a cap-fitted panendoscope for esophagus, stomach, and colon mucosal lesions. *Gastrointest Endosc* 1993; **39**: 58–62.

7 Tanabe S, Koizumi W, Kokutou M *et al.* Usefulness of endoscopic aspiration mucosectomy as compared with strip biopsy for the treatment of gastric mucosal cancer. *Gastrointest Endosc* 1999; **50**: 819–22.

8 Suzuki H. Endoscopic mucosal resection using ligating device for early gastric cancer. *Gastrointest Endosc Clin N Am* 2001; **11**: 511–18.

9 Ono H, Kondo H, Gotoda T *et al.* Endoscopic mucosal resection for treatment of early gastric cancer. *Gut* 2001; **48**: 225–9.

10 Gotoda T, Kondo H, Ono H *et al.* A new endoscopic mucosal resection procedure using an insulation-tipped electrosurgical knife for rectal flat lesions. *Gastrointest Endosc* 1999; **50**: 560–3.

11 Oda I, Gotoda T, Hamanaka H *et al.* Endoscopic submucosal dissection for early gastric cancer: technical feasibility, operation time and complications from a large consecutive series. *Dig Endosc* 2005; **17**: 54–8.

12 Yamamoto H, Kawata H, Sunada K *et al.* Successful one-piece resection of large superficial tumors in the stomach and colon using sodium hyaluronate and small-caliber-tip transparent hood. *Endoscopy* 2003; **35**: 690–4.

13 Oyama T, Kikuchi Y. Aggressive endoscopic mucosal resection in the upper GI tract – hook knife EMR method. *Minim Invasive Ther Allied Technol* 2002; **11**: 291–5.

14 Yahagi N, Fujishiro M, Kakushima N *et al.* Endoscopic submucosal dissection for early gastric cancer using the tip of an electrosurgical snare (thin type). *Dig Endosc* 2004; **16**: 34–8.

15 Gotoda T. Endoscopic resection of early gastric cancer. *Gastric Cancer* 2007; **10**: 1–11.

16 Eguchi T, Gotoda T, Oda I, Hamanaka H, Hasuike N, Saito D. Is endoscopic one-piece mucosal resection essential for early gastric cancer? *Dig. Endosc* 2003; **15**: 113–16.

17 Gotoda T, Yanagisawa A, Sasako M *et al.* Incidence of lymph node metastasis from early gastric cancer: estimation with a large number of cases at two large centers. *Gastric Cancer* 2000; **3**: 219–25.

18 Rosch T, Sarbia M, Schmacher B *et al.* Attempted endoscopic en bloc resection of mucosal and submucosal tumors using insulated-tip knives: a pilot series. *Endoscopy* 2004; **36**: 788–801.

19 Choi IJ, Kim CG, Chang HJ, Kim SG, Kook MC, Bae JM. The learning curve for EMR with circumferential mucosal incision in treating intramucosal gastric cancer. *Gastrointest Endosc* 2005; **62**: 860–5.

20 Hosokawa K, Yoshida S. Recent advances in endoscopic mucosal resection for early gastric cancer [in Japanese with English abstract]. *Jpn J Cancer Chemother* 1998; **25**: 483.

21 Japanese Society for Esophageal Disease. Guidelines for the clinical and pathologic studies for carcinoma of the esophagus. *Jpn J Surg* 1976; **6**: 79–86.

22 Takeshita K, Tani M, Inoue H *et al.* Endoscopic treatment of early oesophageal or gastric cancer. *Gut* 1997; **40**: 123–7.

23 Inoue H. Endoscopic mucosal resection for esophageal and gastric mucosal cancers. *Can J Gastroenterol* 1998; **12**: 355–9.

24 Narahara H, Iishi H, Tatsuta M *et al.* Effectiveness of endoscopic mucosal resection with submucosal saline injection technique for superficial squamous carcinomas of the esophagus. *Gastrointest Endosc* 2000; **52**: 730–4.

25 Araki K, Ohno S, Egashira A, Saeki H, Kawaguchi H, Sugimachi K. Pathologic features of superficial esophageal squamous cell carcinoma with lymph node and distal metastasis. *Cancer* 2002; **94**: 570–5.

26 Shimizu Y, Tsukagoshi H, Fujita M, Hosokawa M, Kato M, Asaka M. Long-term outcome after endoscopic mucosal resection in patients with esophageal squamous cell carcinoma invading the muscularis mucosae or deeper. *Gastrointest Endosc* 2002; **56**: 387–90.

27 Higuchi K, Tanabe S, Koizumi W *et al.* Expansion of the indications for endoscopic mucosal resection in patients with superficial esophageal carcinoma. *Endoscopy* 2007; **39**: 36–40.

28 Pesko P, Rakic S, Milicevic M, Bulajic P, Gerzic Z. Prevalence and clinicopathologic features of multiple squamous cell carcinoma of the esophagus. *Cancer* 1994; **73**: 2687–90.

29 Fujishiro M, Yahagi N, Kakushima N *et al.* Endoscopic submucosal dissection of esophageal squamous cell neoplasms. *Clin Gastroenterol Hepatol* 2006; **4**: 688–94.

30 Ono A, Fujii T, Saito Y *et al.* Endoscopic submucosal resection of rectal carcinoid tumors with a ligation device. *Gastrointest Endosc* 2003; **57**: 583–7.

31 Saito Y, Uraoka T, Matsuda T *et al.* Endoscopic treatment of large superficial colorectal tumors: a case series of 200 endoscopic submucosal dissections (with video). *Gastrointest Endosc* 2007; Epub ahead of print.

32 Yamamoto S, Watanabe M, Hasegawa H *et al.* The risk of lymph node metastasis in T1 colorectal carcinoma. *Hepatogastroenterology* 2004; **51**: 998–1000.

33 Bergmann U, Beger HG. Endoscopic mucosal resection for advanced non-polypoid colorectal adenoma and early stage carcinoma. *Surg Endosc* 2003; **17**: 475–9.

34 Tung SY, Wu CS, Wu MC, Su MY. Endoscopic treatment of colorectal polyps and early cancer. *Dig Dis Sci* 2001; **46**: 1152–6.

35 Zlatanic J, Waye JD, Kim PS, Baiocco PJ, Gleim GW. Large sessile colonic adenomas: use of argon plasma coagulator to supplement piecemeal snare polypectomy. *Gastrointest Endosc* 1999; **49**: 731–5.

36 Brooker JC, Saunders BP, Shah SG, Thapar CJ, Suzuki N, Williams CB. Treatment with argon plasma coagulation reduces recurrence after piecemeal resection of large sessile colonic polyps: a randomized trial and recommendations. *Gastrointest Endosc* 2002; **55**: 371–5.

37 Regula J, Wronska E, Polkowski M *et al.* Argon plasma coagulation after piecemeal polypectomy of sessile colorectal adenomas: long-term follow-up study. *Endoscopy* 2003; **35**: 212–18.

38 Conio M, Repici A, Demarquay JF, Blanchi S, Dumas R, Filiberti R. EMR of large sessile colorectal polyps. *Gastrointest Endosc* 2004; **60**: 234–41.

39 Jameel JK, Pillinger SH, Moncur P, Tsai HH, Duthie GS. Endoscopic mucosal resection (EMR) in the management of large colorectal polyps. *Colorectal Dis* 2006; **8**: 497–500.

40 Saito Y, Fujii T, Kondo H *et al.* Endoscopic treatment for laterally spreading tumors in the colon. *Endoscopy* 2001; **33**: 682–6.

41 Saito Y, Fujii T, Kondo H *et al.* Endoscopic treatment for laterally spreading tumors in the colon. *Endoscopy* 2001; **33**: 682–6.

42 Uraoka T, Saito Y, Matsuda T *et al.* Endoscopic indications for endoscopic mucosal resection of laterally spreading tumours in the colorectum. *Gut* 2006; **55**: 1592–7.

43 Saito Y, Uraoka T, Matsuda T *et al.* A pilot study to assess the safety and efficacy of carbon dioxide insufflation during colorectal endoscopic submucosal dissection with the patient under conscious sedation, *Gastrointest Endosc* 2007; **65**: 537–42.

44 Repici A, Conio M, De Angelis C *et al.* Insulated-tip knife endoscopic mucosal resection of large colorectal polyps unsuitable for standard polypectomy. *Am J Gastroenterol* 2007; **102**: 1617–23.

How to Cope with Complications Throughout the Gastrointestinal Tract

ICHIRO ODA, HISATOMO IKEHARA, CHIZU YOKOI,
TAKAHISA MATSUDA AND PRADEEP BHANDARI

Introduction

Endoscopic resection has been accepted as a less invasive treatment for gastro-intestinal (GI) tumors which have a negligible risk of lymph node metastasis [1–5]. It should be safe, effective, and applicable to a variety of clinical situations. However, there is a risk of complications related to endoscopic resection, which include bleeding, perforation, and stricture formation.

As the number of patients who undergo endoscopic resection increases, the number of complications may increase. The number of patients with early gastric cancer who undergo endoscopic resection is increasing in Japan, because the indications are expanded and the techniques are improving. The general indications of endoscopic resection for early gastric cancer proposed by the Japanese Gastric Cancer Association includes: (1) differentiated adenocarcinoma; (2) intramucosal cancer; (3) ≤20 mm in size; and (4) without ulcer findings [6]. Early gastric cancer which can be treated under these criteria is limited to small tumors without ulcer findings, allowing one-piece resection by conventional endoscopic mucosal resection (EMR) [7–10]. Recently the indications for endoscopic resection for early gastric cancer have been expanded, based on the risks of lymph node metastasis in early gastric cancer obtained from a large number of surgical cases [6,11]. The expanded indications include lesions ≥20 mm and ulcerative lesions which were originally resected by surgery. The new technique of endoscopic submucosal dissection (ESD) has been developed to obtain one-piece resection during endoscopic resection for even large and ulcerative lesions [12–17].

Endoscopic Mucosal Resection. Edited by M. Conio, P. Siersema, A. Repici and T. Ponchon. © 2008 Blackwell Publishing. ISBN 978-1-4051-5885-5.

In other GI tumors, as the improvement of diagnostic techniques such as chromoendoscopy, high magnification endoscopy, and narrow band imaging can facilitate early detection, the number of patients who undergo endoscopic resection may increase.

Consequently, physicians must be able to treat patients who have complications related to endoscopic resection. In this chapter, we describe how to cope with complications throughout the gastrointestinal tract.

Stomach

Perforation

Incidence
Perforation is uncommon with EMR techniques [18], but in ESD has been reported as about 4% of gastric wall perforations [17]. We have reported the rate of gastric perforation according to lesion location, size, and ulcer finding (Table 14.1) [17,19]. The rates of gastric perforation in the upper and middle third of the stomach, especially the greater curvature of the gastric body, are higher than in the lower third of the stomach, probably because the gastric wall in these locations is comparatively thin. The endoscopic procedure for lesions on the upper and middle third of the stomach had to be achieved with a retroflexed view, compared to that of a straight view for the lesions on the lower third of the stomach. The rates of gastric perforation in larger lesions and ulcerative lesions are higher than in smaller lesions and non-ulcerative lesions.

Table 14.1 Relationship between gastric wall perforation induced by ESD and lesion location, size, and ulcer finding [17].

	Perforation	*p* value
Location		
U	7% (13/176)	
M	4% (16/431)	<0.001
L	1% (6/426)	<0.05
Size (mm)		
≤20	3% (18/719)	
21–30	3% (6/176)	
≥31	8% (11/138)	0.001
Ulcer finding		
Positive	6% (14/243)	<0.005
Negative	3% (21/790)	

U: upper third; M: middle third; L: lower third.

Prevention

The potential mechanisms of perforation induced by EMR and proposed techniques to avoid it are reported as follows: (1) Inadequate amount of submucosal injection and/or excessively large snare being used; (2) consequently, when the snare is closed, excessive tissue will be grasped. One way of detecting this problem is to move the snare back and forth. If the muscularis propria is entrapped, the whole wall, as opposed to only the lesion, may be seen to move; and (3) slightly loosening the grasp of the snare while tenting the mucosa into the lumen and toward the endoscope may help to release potentially entrapped muscularis propria. Alternating forward and backward movements of the snare are also often performed to avoid entrapment of the muscularis propria. The closed snare then captures a smaller amount of tissue. If there is still uncertainty about whether there is entrapment of the muscularis propria, the loop is fully opened, and repeat snaring with or without repeat submucosal injection is performed [3].

The perforation induced by ESD usually occurs a process of submucosal dissection not of circumferential incision. The potential mechanisms of perforation induced by ESD are submucosal dissection with less space in the submucosal layer and misunderstanding of the gastric wall curve. Figure. 14.1 shows a moment of preparation. The IT knife goes to the muscle layer. To avoid this, adequate space in the submucosal layer between the muscularis propria and the mucosal layer is indispensable. For that purpose, an adequate amount of submucosal injection is necessary. To keep lifting the mucosa for a longer period, the use of sodium hyaluronate, Glyceol, or a mixture of sodium hyaluronate and

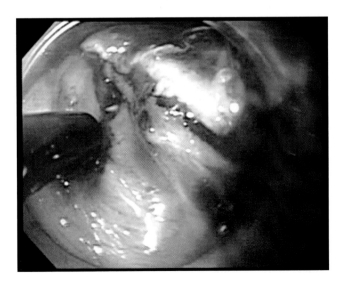

Fig. 14.1 The potential mechanism of perforation induced by ESD is misunderstanding of the gastric wall curve during submucosal dissection.

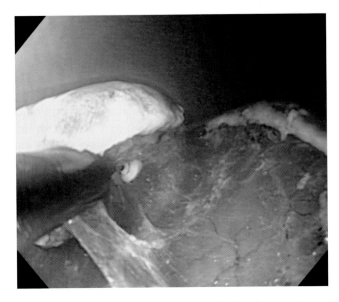

Fig. 14.2   Fluid solution for submucosal injection is mixed with indigo carmine to distinguish the white muscularis propria from the blue submucosal layer.

Glyceol for submucosal injection has been reported as effective [15,20–23]. Special knives such as an insulation-tipped (IT) knife (KD-610L; Olympus Medical Systems Corp., Tokyo, Japan), Hook knife (KD-620-L; Olympus Medical Systems Corp., Tokyo, Japan), and Flex knife (KD-630L; Olympus Medical Systems Corp., Tokyo, Japan) are useful to keep the space from the muscularis propria (see Chapter 7, Fig. 7.3(a)–(c)). We can make the space by the ceramic ball of the tip of the IT knife, by the pulling hook knife and by the thick tip of the sheath of the flex knife. The use of fluid solution mixed with indigo carmine for submucosal injection is effective for recognizing the gastric wall curve. We can distinguish the white muscularis propria from the blue submucosal layer (Fig. 14.2). The use of transparent attachment of the scope is also useful. We can recognize the gastric wall curve by lifting the mucosal layer using the attachment.

Management

Endoscopic closure.   In the past, when gastric perforation occurred during endoscopic resection, emergency surgery was usually performed and the merits of the resection were lost [19]. Endoscopic closure of a perforation by using clips after snare excision of a gastric leiomyoma, was first reported by Binmoeller *et al.* [24] in 1993. The metallic clips were originally developed for hemostatic purposes [25].

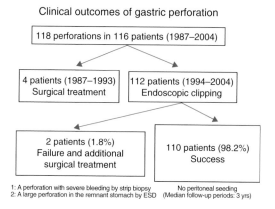

Clinical outcomes of gastric perforation

118 perforations in 116 patients (1987–2004)

4 patients (1987–1993) Surgical treatment

112 patients (1994–2004) Endoscopic clipping

2 patients (1.8%) Failure and additional surgical treatment

110 patients (98.2%) Success

1: A perforation with severe bleeding by strip biopsy   No peritoneal seeding
2: A large perforation in the remnant stomach by ESD   (Median follow-up periods: 3 yrs)

Fig. 14.3 The results of 121 patients with gastric perforation during endoscopic resections for early gastric cancer [118].

We also used a non-surgical treatment such as endoscopic closure with endoclips as a less invasive method of the treatment of gastric perforations after endoscopic resection and reported that it proved useful [19]. The results of 116 patients with gastric perforation during endoscopic resections for early gastric cancer are shown in Fig. 14.3. The initial four patients, who underwent endoscopic resection from 1987 to 1993 were treated by emergent surgery. In 110 patients (98.2%) among the remaining 112 patients, endoscopic closure was possible and the clinical courses of the patients were favorable under antibiotic therapy with a second-generation cephalosporin.

Two methods of endoscopic closure are reported: a 'single-closure method' and an 'omental-patch method' using endoclips with a right-angled hook (HX-600-090 or HX-610-090; Olympus Medical Systems Corp., Tokyo, Japan) [19]. A single-closure method is done to treat small defects. The knack for the single-closure method is to start clipping from the edge of the hole not from the center. A perforation hole induced by ESD is smaller and move lined compared to that of a strip biopsy, so a single-closure method can be applied to treat perforations caused by ESD. The knack for closure of defects by ESD is to make enough space for clipping, because perforation by ESD usually occurs in the process of submucosal dissection. An omental-patch method is performed for comparatively larger defects by using either the greater omentum or the lesser omentum as a patch [19].

Peritoneal tap. Vital signs such as blood pressure, oxygen saturation, and electrocardiograms must continuously be checked during these endoscopic procedures. If abdominal fullness because of air leakage from the perforated lesion is severe, breathing deterioration or neurogenic shock can occur. To prevent

Methods	Days
Drip infusion	2–3
Nasogastric tube	1
Antibiotics	2
Fasting	2
Admission period	4–7

Table 14.2 Management after endoscopic clipping for gastric perforation [19].

these complications when gastric perforation occurs, frequent abdominal palpation is recommended to check the degree of abdominal fullness with air. If severe abdominal fullness is noted, decompression of the pneumoperitoneum must be performed with a 14- or 16-gauge puncture needle with side slits. Before puncture, we tested with a 23-gauge needle syringe filled with local anesthetic [19].

Management after endoscopic closure. The management after successful endoscopic closure is shown in Table 14.2. Patients are treated with a nasogastric tube for one day, antibiotics for two days, and start eating after one to two days of fasting [19].

Bleeding

Incidence

Procedure-related bleeding is one of the most common complications. The rates of bleeding have been reported as 1.2–20.5%, which probably vary according to the definition [8,17,18,26–28].

Procedure-related bleeding can be subdivided into immediate bleeding during procedure and delayed bleeding after the procedure from the point of view of time, although there are a few reports in which bleeding was investigated with the definition as immediate and delayed bleeding. Immediate bleeding is not generally frequent with EMR techniques. On the other hand, it is quite common with ESD techniques, and the management for it is indispensable to completion of ESD. We estimated immediate bleeding in terms of a difference in hemoglobin (Hb) level between pre-procedure and next-day values and a diminution of ≥ 2 g/dl in Hb level was defined as significant. Evidence of immediate bleeding was found in 7% [17]. The rates of it in the upper and the middle third of the stomach are higher than in the lower third of the stomach (Table 14.3), probably because the diameter of submucosal arteries in the upper and the middle third of the stomach are significantly larger than that for arteries in the lower third of the stomach.

The rate of delayed bleeding after EMR reported from various institutions is 5.3% [28]. Delayed bleeding after ESD was reported as 6% [17]. The rates of it in the lower and the middle third of the stomach are higher than in the upper

Table 14.3 Relationship between immediate bleeding during gastric endoscopic submucosal dissection and lesion location, size, and ulcer finding [17].

	Diminution of Hb level ($\geq$2 g/dl)*	p value
Location		
U	8% (14/176)	0.01
M	8% (35/431)	<0.005
L	3% (14/426)	
Size (mm)		
$\leq$20	4% (32/719)	0.065
21–30	8% (14/176)	
$\geq$31	12% (17/138)	<0.001
Ulcer finding		
Positive	7% (17/243)	0.504
Negative	6% (46/790)	

U: upper third; M: middle third; L: lower third.
* Immediate bleeding was estimated in terms of a difference of Hb level between pre-procedure and next-day values.

Table 14.4 Relationship between delayed bleeding after gastric endoscopic submucosal dissection and lesion location, size, ulcer finding, and time since procedure [17].

	Delayed bleeding	p value
Location		
U	1% (1/176)	
M	6% (27/431)	0.001
L	6% (31/426)	<0.001
Size (mm)		
$\leq$20	5% (35/719)	
21–30	7% (13/176)	0.1838
$\geq$31	8% (11/138)	0.1385
Ulcer finding		
Positive	5% (13/243)	
Negative	6% (46/790)	0.7811
Time		
$\leq$24 h	76% (45/59)	
2–7 days	12% (7/59)	
8–15 days	12% (7/59)	

U: upper third; M: middle third; L: lower third.

third of the stomach (Table 14.4), again probably because the diameter of submucosal arteries in the upper and the middle third of the stomach were significantly larger than that for arteries in the lower third of the stomach. The reason for the latter remains unclear but antral peristaltic activity may contribute to this to some extent. It is also speculated that this increase in the risk of bleeding from lesions of the lower third of the stomach could be due to the fact that intra-operative bleeding in this group of lesions is low, and therefore needs less intra-operative hemostatic treatment compared to vessels in the lesions of the upper third of the stomach. This lack of intra-operative intervention may contribute toward the risk of delayed bleeding.

Management

Acid suppressing drug.   In general, proton pump inhibitors are used for acid suppressing for two months. Their use is based on the observation that the stability of a blood clot is reduced in an acid environment. Thus a pH greater than 6 is necessary for platelet aggregation while clot lysis occurs when the pH falls below 6. There are no convincing data to support the use of H2 receptor antagonists, and these drugs do not reliably or consistently increase gastric pH to 6 [29].

Endoscopic treatment modality.   Endoscopic treatment modalities for GI tract bleeding are divided into cautery, injection methods, and mechanical therapy. Cautery devices include heat probes, argon plasma coagulation (APC), and electrocautery forceps, and so on. The method of action of injection therapy is primary tamponade because of volume effect, with some agents having a secondary pharmacologic effect. The types of the solution include normal saline with epinephrine (of which the main mechanism is tamponade), hypertonic sodium chloride with epinephrine (which has both primary tamponade and secondary direct tissue injury and thrombosis), and ethanol (of which the main mechanism is direct tissue injury and thrombosis). The mechanical therapy refers to the implantation of a device that causes physical tamponade of a bleeding site. Currently, the only mechanical therapies widely available are endoscopically placed clips and band ligation devices. Endoscopic clips are usually placed over a bleeding site (e.g. visible vessel) and left in place. Endoscopic band ligation devices, commonly used in variceal bleeding, have also been used to treat nonvariceal causes of bleeding and involve the placement of elastic bands over tissue to produce mechanical compression and tamponade.

Hemostasis for immediate bleeding.   Cautery is used for hemostasis against immediate bleeding during endoscopic resection, because clips disturb the following resection. We usually use electrocautery using different devices according to the degree of bleeding. Minor oozing bleeding can be controlled by cautery using a cutting device such as a needle knife, IT knife, Hook knife, or Flex knife. Electro-Surgical Unit (ESU) is set up as 50 W of Forced coagulation mode (ICC200; ERBE Corp., Tubingen, Germany) or 50 W, Effect 5 of Swift coagulation mode (VIO 300D; ERBE Corp., Tubingen, Germany) for this cautery. It is necessary to pre-coagulate for prevention of bleeding using a cutting device with the same setting of ESU, when vessels are found. Cautery using hemostatic forceps such as Coagrasper (FD-410LR; Olympus Medical Systems Corp., Tokyo, Japan) or hot biopsy forceps (Radial Jaw; Boston Scientific Corp., Natick, Mass.) are suitable for massive bleeding. ESU is set up as 80W of Soft coagulation mode (ICC200; ERBE Corp., Tubingen, Germany) or 80W, Effect 5 of Soft coagulation mode (VIO 300D; ERBE Corp., Tubingen, Germany) for this cautery. The knack for hemostasis is to find the exact bleeding point by water flash and take aim at it.

Hemostasis for delayed bleeding.   All sorts of the abovementioned endoscopic treatment modalities can be used in combination or on their own for hemostasis against delayed bleeding after endoscopic resection. We use different modalities according to the period of bleeding. In the early days of delayed bleeding, the artificial ulcer floor is still soft with less granulation tissue, so endoscopic clips or electrocautery using hemostatic forceps can be applied. In the latter days of delayed bleeding, the artificial ulcer floor is getting hard with granulation tissue, so injection method using a solution that has direct tissue injury and thrombosisis is preferred. In our series, 76% of patients bled within 24 hours and the remaining 24% bled between 2 and 15 days after the procedure (Table 14.4) [17].

Stenosis

Incidence
Bleeding and perforation remain major complications. Stenosis after endoscopic resection for lesions located near cardia or the pylorus is an important late complication, as it results in severe dysphagia. A total of 2011 early gastric cancers resected by ESD between 2000 and 2005 were reviewed at our institution. These were located at the upper third of the stomach in 326 lesions, the middle third in 887 lesions, and the lower third in 798 lesions. The resections in which mucosal defects included squamo-columnar junction (SCJ resection) were found in 41 of the 326 upper third lesions. The resections in which mucosal defects included pylorus ring (pylorus resection) were found in 115 of the 798 lower third lesions. Significant stenosis was defined as present when a standard 11 mm diameter endoscope (GIF Q240, Q230, Q200, Olympus Medical Systems Corp., Tokyo, Japan) could not be passed through the stricture. Significant stenosis developed in seven (17%) of the 41 SCJ resections and eight (7%) of the 115 pylorus resections after ESD (Tables 14.5 and 14.6). There was a significant relationship between degree of luminal circumferential mucosal defect and the development of significant stenosis. There

Table 14.5 Circumferential mucosal defect and stenosis after
endoscopic submucosal dissection in the pylorus resection*

Grade of circumferential mucosal defect	Stenosis	p value
–1/2	0% (0/81)	
1/2–3/4	0% (0/16)	
3/4–	44% (8/18)	<0.001
Total	7% (8/115)	

*Pylorus resection was defined as resection in which mucosal defects included
pylorus ring.

Table 14.6 Circumferential mucosal defect and stenosis after
ESD in the SCJ resection*

Grade of circumferential mucosal defect	Stenosis	p value
~1/2	0% (0/28)	
1/2–3/4	0% (0/6)	
3/4–	100% (7/7)	<0.001
Total	17% (7/41)	

*SCJ resection was defined as resection in which mucosal defects included
squamo-columnar junction.

was no stenosis in the 34 SCJ resections and 97 pylorus resections in which
mucosal defects after ESD were less than three-quarters of the luminal circumference. On the other hand, all (100%) of the seven SCJ resections in which
mucosal defects after ESD were over three-quarters of the luminal circumference developed stenosis, and eight (44%) of the 18 pylorus resections after
ESD over three-quarters of the luminal circumference developed stenosis.

Bleeding and perforation are complications that usually occur during
endoscopic resection or within 24 h of the procedure and thus treatment is
usually immediate. In contrast, stenosis manifests a few weeks after endoscopic
resection during the healing process. In our series, the median period between
ESD and the first endoscopic dilatation was 22 days in the patients with significant stenosis in SCJ resections and 30 days in the pylorus resections.

Management
If a patient with significant stenosis complains of dysphagia, endoscopic
dilatation is performed with a 15–18 mm balloon dilator (CRE Wireguided

Balloon Dilatation Catheter; Boston Scientific Corp., Natick, Mass.). Dilation is continued until dysphagia resolves. In our series, dysphagia and significant stenosis fully resolved in all patients in response to repeated balloon dilatation. The median frequencies of repeated balloon dilatation were five times in the patients with significant stenosis in SCJ resections and nine times in the pylorus resections. The median periods of repeated balloon dilatation were 42 days in the patients with significant stenosis in SCJ resections and 52 days in the pylorus resections.

Colon

Most therapeutic colonoscopies are done in the outpatient clinic without hospital admission excluding endoscopic resection for large tumors. Familiarity with the endoscopic findings, symptoms and signs of complications, and treatment of complications is a prerequisite for performance of colonoscopic polypectomy and mucosal resection.

Perforation

During therapeutic colonoscopy, perforation is the most serious accidental disorder and requires rapid and appropriate management [30–33]. The rate of perforations due to therapeutic colonoscopies has varied from 0.1% to 0.85%, while mortality has ranged from 0.01% to 0.34% [30–37]. Taku *et al.* [37] reported the rate of perforation according to the methods of therapeutic colonoscopies. The overall rate of occurrence of perforation was 0.15% (23/15 160). Perforation rate for EMR (0.58%) showed a significantly higher rate ($p < 0.0001$) than that for hot biopsy and polypectomy. The rate for ESD (14%) showed a markedly higher rate ($p < 0.0001$) than that for other standard procedures.

   Generally, surgery is the first choice of treatment, because it is difficult to manage chemical or bacterial peritonitis due to intraperitoneal leakage of intestinal fluid containing chemical substances such as digestive enzymes, and fecal fluid containing large amounts of bacteria via the perforated site [30–39]. Patients who developed sepsis and died of peritonitis due to delayed initiation of surgery have also been reported [40]. However, recent reports have suggested the usefulness of endoscopic clipping to prevent leakage of intestinal contents in patients with perforation associated with endoscopic treatment [37,40–46]. Taku *et al.* [37] have reported the indications for endoscopic clipping for perforations during therapeutic colonoscopy as follows: (1) The dimension of the defect is less than 10 mm; (2) adequate bowel preparation was performed; and (3) the patient is in a stable condition after immediate perforation.

Bleeding

Bleeding is the most common complication associated with therapeutic colonoscopies including hot biopsy, snare polypectomy, and endoscopic mucosal resection. The reported incidence varies according to the definition of bleeding, and the size and type of lesions resected. The overall risk is approximately 1–2% for snare polypectomy [47]. Rosen *et al.* [48] reported an 0.4% risk of bleeding requiring hospital admission in a retrospective study involving 4721 patients who had polypectomies. Nivatvongs reported 10 episodes of bleeding requiring blood transfusions among 1172 patients [49]. Binmoeller *et al.* [50] reported a 24% risk of bleeding in a series of 176 large (>3 cm) polypectomies. Most of these hemorrhages occurred during the procedure, and all were successfully treated by endoscopic methods.

Bleeding can occur immediately after the procedure or can be delayed. Immediate bleeding after endoscopic removal is usually a slow ooze, and arterial bleeding is rarely encountered. Almost all of the immediate bleeding could be managed endoscopically with an injection of saline containing epinephrine or by hemoclips, and so on. On the other hand, delayed bleeding is important because of the necessity of repeated colonoscopy or hospitalization. Fu *et al.* [51] have reported the risk factor and clinical course of delayed bleeding after endoscopic resection. The size of the removed lesions was a significant risk factor of delayed bleeding.

A variety of techniques are useful. These include application of the endoclip or endoloop, use of APC, injection of diluted epinephrine, cauterization using monopolar or bipolar instruments, and repeat application of the snare or hot-forceps biopsy to grasp the remnant stalk of pedunculated polyp [47,52]. In cases of delayed bleeding, we typically would purge the bowel using 4 to 6L of polyethylene glycol solution within three hours, immediately followed by a colonoscopy [47]. On the other hand, Rex and colleagues have reported successful colonoscopic treatment of delayed post-polypectomy bleeding without prior bowel purge [53].

Esophagus

Perforation

The reported rates of perforation induced by EMR in the esophagus are 1.4–2.5% [54,55].

Although there are few reports of perforations caused by endoscopic resection in the esophagus, esophageal perforations caused by balloon dilation are described; the management of such cases is highly controversial. Some surgeons recommend early surgical treatment [56–58], whereas others recommend consideration of conservative therapy [59–61].

Shimizu *et al.* [55] have reported three cases of successful closures of esophageal perforations after EMR with endoscopically applied clips. In their opinion, closure of esophageal perforations from EMR by endoscopic clip application is appropriate therapy if the perforation is recognized immediately and is not larger than 1–1.5 cm in shortest diameter. When this method of treatment is used, the patient must be observed for an extended period of time, with particular attention to signs of a transition from localized inflammation to generalized mediastinitis.

Bleeding

Kodama *et al.* [62] have described a bleeding rate (1.5%, 6/396) of EMR for patients with superficial esophageal cancer in the survey of Japanese institutions.

A variety of techniques are useful for bleeding of esophageal EMR. These include application of the endoclip, use of APC and cauterization using monopolar or bipolar instruments.

Stenosis

Esophageal stenosis after endoscopic resection is an important late complication, as it results in severe dysphagia. In particular, large mucosal defects are more likely to lead to stricture formation in the esophagus because the lumen is much narrower than in the stomach and the colon. Esophageal stenosis developed after EMR has been described by Katada *et al.* [63]. Significant stenosis was defined as present when a standard 11 mm diameter endoscope (GIF Q240, Q230, Q200, Olympus Optical Co. Ltd., Tokyo, Japan) could not be passed through the stricture. It was found in 13 (6.0%) of 216 superficial esophageal lesions. In all these cases endoscopic mucosal resection resulted in a mucosal defect that involved over three-quarters of the luminal circumference. There was a significant relationship between degree of luminal circumferential mucosal defect and the development of significant stenosis. There was no stenosis in the 197 resections with mucosal defects involving less than three-quarters of the luminal circumference. On the other hand, 13 (68%) of the 19 resections involving over three-quarters of the luminal circumference developed stenosis. There was also a significant relationship between longitudinal length of the mucosal defect and the development of esophageal stenosis. The esophageal stenosis was more frequent in the subgroup of patients with mucosal defects involving over three-quarters of the circumference, those with a mucosal defect over 30 mm long (10/10; 100%) compared to those with a mucosal defect less than 30 mm long (3/9; 33%).

All patients with esophageal stenosis experienced dysphagia and all therefore required endoscopic balloon dilatation. The dysphagia fully resolved in all patients with esophageal stenosis in response to repeated balloon dilatation. A total of 85 balloon dilatations were performed (median 5 per patient, range 1–15). In the subgroup of patients with mucosal defects involving over three-quarters of the circumference, those with a mucosal defect over 30 mm long required more frequent balloon dilatation (mean 8 [4.3] times), and the stenosis was of longer duration (mean 16 [17.7] months) than those with defects 30 mm or less in length (respectively, 1 [0.6] times and 2 [1.9] months).

References

1 Rembacken BJ, Gotoda T, Fujii T et al. Endoscopic mucosal resection. Endoscopy 2001; 33: 709–18.
2 Ponchon T. Endoscopic mucosal resection. J Clin Gastroenterol. 200l; 32: 6–10.
3 Soetikno R, Gotoda T, Nakanishi Y et al. Endoscopic mucosal resection. Gastrointest Endosc 2003; 57: 567–79.
4 Soetikno R, Kaltenbach T, Yeh Rd, Gotoda T. Endoscopic mucosal resection for early cancers of the upper gastrointestinal tract. J Clin Oncol 2005; 23: 4490–8.
5 Conio M, Ponchon T, Blanchi S, Filiberti R. Endoscopic mucosal resection. Am J Gastroenterol 2006; 101: 653–63.
6 Eguchi T, Gotoda T, Oda I et al. Is endoscopic one-piece mucosal resection essential for early gastric cancer? Dig Endosc 2003; 15: 113–16.
7 Tada M, Murakami A, Karita M et al. Endoscopic resection of early gastric cancer. Endoscopy 1993; 25: 445–51.
8 Tanabe S, Koizumi W, Kokutou M et al. Usefulness of endoscopic aspiration mucosectomy as compared with strip biopsy for the treatment of gastric mucosal cancer. Gastrointest Endosc 1999; 50: 819–22.
9 Inoue H, Takeshita K, Hori H et al. Endoscopic mucosal resection with a cap-fitted panendoscope for esophagus, stomach, and colon mucosal lesions. Gastrointest Endosc 1993; 39: 58–62.
10 Tanabe S, Koizumi W, Mitomi H et al. Clinical outome of endoscopic aspiration mucosectomy for early gastric cancer. Gastrointest Endosc 2002; 56: 708–13.
11 Gotoda T, Yanagisawa A, Sasako M et al. Incidence of lymph node metastasis from early gastric cancer: estimation with a large number of cases at two large centers. Gastric Cancer 2000; 3: 219–25.
12 Hirao M, Masuda K, Asanuma T et al. Endoscopic resection of early gastric cancer and other tumors with local injection of hypertonic saline-epinephrine. Gastrointest Endosc 1988; 34: 264–9.
13 Ono H, Kondo H, Gotoda T et al. Endoscopic mucosal resection for treatment of early gastric cancer. Gut 2001; 48: 225–9.
14 Gotoda T, Kondo H, Ono H et al. A new endoscopic mucosal resection procedure using an insulation-tipped electrosurgical knife for rectal flat lesions. Gastrointest Endosc 1999; 50: 560–3.
15 Yamamoto H, Kawata H, Sunada K et al. Successful one-piece resection of large superficial tumors in the stomach and colon using sodium hyaluronate and small-caliber-tip transparent hood. Endoscopy 2003; 35: 690–4.

16 Oyama T, Kikuchi Y. Aggressive endoscopic mucosal resection in the upper GI tract – Hook knife EMR method. *Min Invas Ther & Allied Technol* 2002; **11**: 291–5.

17 Oda I, Gotoda T, Hamanaka H *et al.* Endoscopic submucosal dissection for early gastric cancer: technical feasibility, operation time and complications from a large consecutive series. *Dig Endosc* 2005; **17**: 54–8.

18 Kojima T, Parra-Blanco A, Takahashi H *et al.* Outcome of endoscopic mucosal resection for early gastric cancer: review of the Japanese literature. *Gastrointest Endosc* 1998; **48**: 550–4.

19 Minami S, Gotoda T, Ono H, Oda I, Hamanaka H. Complete endoscopic closure of gastric perforation induced by endoscopic resection of early gastric cancer using endoclips can prevent surgery (with video). *Gastrointest Endosc* 2006; **63**: 596–601.

20 Jin Hyun J, Rae Chun H, Jai Chun H *et al.* Comparison of the characteristics of submucosal injection solutions used in endoscopic mucosal resection. *Scand J Gastroenterol* 2006; **41**: 488–92.

21 Fujishiro M, Yahagi N, Kashimura K *et al* Comparison of various submucosal injection solutions for maintaining mucosal elevation during endoscopic mucosal resection. *Endoscopy* 2004; **36**: 579–83.

22 Uraoka T, Fujii T, Saito Y *et al.* Effectiveness of glycerol as a submucosal injection for EMR. *Gastrointest Endosc* 2005; **61**: 736–40.

23 Fujishiro M, Yahagi N, Kashimura K *et al* Tissue damage of different submucosal injection solutions for EMR. *Gastrointest Endosc* 2005; **62**: 933–42.

24 Binmoeller KF, Grimm H, Soehendra N. Endoscopic closure of a perforation using metallic clips after snare excision of gastric leiomyoma. *Gastrointest Endosc* 1993; **39**: 172–4.

25 Hachisu T. Evaluation of endoscopic hemostasis using an improved clipping apparatus. *Surg Endosc* 1988; **2**: 13–17.

26 Ida K, Nakazawa S, Yoshino J *et al.* Multicentre collaborative prospective study of endoscopic treatment of early gastric cancer. *Diges Endosc* 2004; **16**: 295–302.

27 Shiba M, Higuchi K, Kadouchi K *et al.* Risk factors for bleeding after endoscopic mucosal resection. *World J Gastroenterol* 2005; **46**: 7335–9.

28 Okano A, Hajiro K, Takakuwa H *et al.* Predictors of bleeding after endoscopic mucosal resection of gastric tumors. *Gastrointest Endosc* 2003; **57**: 687–90.

29 British Society of Gastroenterology Endoscopy Committee. Non-variceal upper gastrointestinal haemorrhage: guidelines. *Gut* 2002; **51(Suppl IV)**: iv1–6.

30 Kavin H, Sinicrope F, Esker AH. Management of perforation of the colon at colonoscopy. *Am J Gastroenterol* 1992; **87**: 161–7.

31 Farley DR, Bannon MP, Zietlow SP *et al.* Management of colonoscopic perforations. *Mayo Clin Proc* 1992; **72**: 729–33.

32 Waye JD, Kahn O, Auerbach ME. Complications of colonoscopy and flexible sigmoidoscopy. *Gastrointest Endosc Clin N Am* 1996; **6**: 343–77.

33 Putcha RV, Burdick JS. Management of iatrogenic perforation. *Gastroenterol Clin North Am* 2003; **32**: 1289–1309.

34 Orsoni P, Berdah S, Verrier C *et al.* Colonic perforation due to colonoscopy: a retrospective study of 48 cases. *Endoscopy* 1997; **29**: 160–4.

35 Anderson ML, Pasha TM, Leighton JA. Endoscopic perforation of the colon: lessons from a 10-year study. *Am J Gastroenterol* 2000; **95**: 3418–3422.

36 Kaneko E, Harada H, Kasugai T *et al. Gastroenterol Endosc* 2000; **42**: 308–13 [in Japanese].

37 Taku K, Sano Y, Fu KI *et al.* Iatrogenic perforation associated with therapeutic colonoscopy: a multicenter study in Japan. *J Gastroenterol Hepatol* 2007; **22**: 1409–1414.

38 Lo AY, Beaton HL. Selective management of colonoscopic perforations. *J Am Coll Surg* 1994; **179**: 333–7.

39 Hall C, Dorricott NJ, Donovan IA, Neoptolemos JP. Colon perforation during colonoscopy: surgical versus conservative management. *Br J Surg* 1991; **78**: 542–4.

40 Soliman A, Grundman M. Conservative management of colonoscopic perforation can be misleading. *Endoscopy* 1998; **30**: 790–2.

41 Yshikane H, Hidano H, Sakakibara A *et al.* Endoscopic repair by clipping of iatrogenic colonic perforation. *Gastrointest Endosc* 1997; **46**: 464–6.

42 Kaneko T, Akamatsu T, Shimodaira K *et al.* Nonsurgical treatment of duodenal perforation by endoscopic repair using a clipping device. *Gastrointest Endosc* 1999; **50:** 410–13.

43 Yoshikane H, Hidano H, Sakakibara A *et al.* Feasibility study on endoscopic suture with the combination of a distal attachment and a rotatable clip for complications of endoscopic resection in the large intestine. *Endoscopy* 2000; **32:** 477–80.

44 Baron TH, Gostout CJ, Herman L. Hemoclip repair of a sphincterotomy-induced duodenal perforation. *Gastrointest Endosc* 2000; **52:** 566–8.

45 Mana F, De Vogelaere K, Urban D. Iatrogenic perforation of the colon during diagnostic colonoscopy: endoscopic treatment with clips. Gastrointest Endosc 2001; **54:** 258–9.

46 Fu KI, Sano Y, Sigeharu K *et al.* Colonic perforation after endoscopic biopsy of a submucosal tumor: successful conservative treatment. *Dig Endosc* 2002; **14:** 181–3.

47 Soetikno R, Friedland S, Matsuda T, Gotoda T. (2005) Colonoscopic polypectomy and mucosal resection. In: Ginsberg GG, Kochman ML, Norton I, Gostout CJ, eds. *Clinical Gastrointestinal Endoscopy.* Elsevier Saunders, Philadelphia, 2005: 549–68.

48 Rosen L, Bub DS, Reed JF 3rd, Nastasee SA. Hemorrhage following colonoscopic polypectomy. *Dis Colon Rectum* 1993; **36:** 1126–31.

49 Nivatvongs S. Complications in colonoscopic polypectomy. An experience with 1,555 polypectomies. *Dis Colon Rectum* 1986; **29:** 825–30.

50 Binmoeller KF, Bohnacker S, Seifert H *et al.* Endoscopic snare excision of 'giant' colorectal polyps. *Gastrointest Endosc* 1996; **43:** 183–8.

51 Fu KI, Sano Y, Kato S *et al.* Is the colonoscopic day surgery feasible? A retrospective analysis of the delayed post resection bleeding cases associated with the therapeutic colonoscopies for colorectal lesions larger than 10 mm. *Gastrointest Endosc* 2002; **55:** pAB27.

52 Parra-Blanco A, Kaminaga N, Kojima T *et al.* Hemoclipping for postpolypectomy and postbiopsy colonic bleeding. *Gastrointest Endosc* 2000; **51:** 37–41.

53 Rex DK, Lewis BS, Waye JD. Colonoscopy and endoscopic therapy for delayed post-polypectomy hemorrhage. *Gastrointest Endosc* 1992; **38:** 127–9.

54 Inoue H, Tani M, Nagai K *et al.* Treatment of esophageal and gastric tumors. *Endoscopy* 1999; **31:** 47–55.

55 Shimizu Y, Kato M, Yamamoto J *et al.* Endoscopic clip application for closure of esophageal perforations caused by EMR. *Gastrointest Endosc* 2004; **60:** 636–9.

56 Slater G, Sicular AA. Esophageal perforation after forceful dilatation in achalasia. *Am Surg* 1982; **195:** 186–8.

57 Brewer LA, Carter R, Mulder GA, Stiles QR. Operations in the management of the perforation of the esophagus. *Am J Surg* 1986; **152:** 62–9.

58 Jones WG II, Ginsberg RJ. Esophageal perforation: a continuing challenge. *Ann Thorac Surg* 1992; **53:** 534–43.

59 Richter JE, Castell DO. (1990) Balloon dilatation for the treatment of achalasia. In: Bennet JR, Hunt RH, eds. *Therapeutic Endoscopy and Radiology of the Gut,* 2nd edn. Springer-Verlag, New York: 82–4.

60 Pasricha PJ, Fleischer DE, Kalloo AN. Endoscopic perforations of the upper digestive tract: a review of their pathogenesis, prevention, and management. *Gastroenterology* 1994; **106:** 787–802.

61 Wewalka FW, Clodi PH, Haidinger D. Endoscopic clipping of esophageal perforation after pneumatic dilatation for achalasia. *Endoscopy* 1995; **27:** 608–11.

62 Kodama M, Kakegawa T. Treatment of superficial cancer of the esophagus: a summary of responses to a questionnaire on superficial cancer of the esophagus in Japan. *Surgery* 1998; **123:** 432–9.

63 Katada C, Muto M, Manabe T *et al.* Esophageal stenosis after endoscopic mucosal resection of superficial esophageal lesions. *Gastrointest Endosc* 2003; **57:** 165–9.

CHAPTER 15

Prototypes and Future Directions of Endoscopic Research

PAUL SWAIN AND KEIICHI IKEDA

Introduction

The advent of endoscopic submucosal dissection (ESD) has expanded the indications for the endoscopic treatment of early gastric cancer and has enabled en bloc resection of larger lesions than before. However, in order to accomplish ESD in safety from beginning to end when a complete en bloc specimen is removed for histological analysis, a skilled and meticulous technique is needed. From the risk management point of view, various devices and scopes for ESD have been developed to facilitate the difficult procedures of ESD and to minimize complication rates.

First, this chapter describes a new ESD technique using two newly developed therapeutic endoscopes, and then endoscopic full-thickness resection (EFTR) is presented as a potential future technique to treat early gastrointestinal cancer.

Endoscope development

Multibending endoscope ('M-scope')

The multibending endoscope, the 'M-scope' (XGIF-2T240M; Olympus Medical Systems, Tokyo, Japan; Fig. 15.1(a),(b)) has two independently bending segments: the proximal section can be deflected in one plane (up/down); the distal section can be deflected in two planes (up/down, right/left), similar to a conventional gastrointestinal (GI) endoscope [1]. A combined operation of these segments allows operators to obtain a variety of visual fields, to selectively approach or recede from the lesions, and to obtain *en face* views, which may

---

Endoscopic Mucosal Resection. Edited by M. Conio, P. Siersema, A. Repici and T. Ponchon. © 2008 Blackwell Publishing. ISBN 978-1-4051-5885-5.

(a)

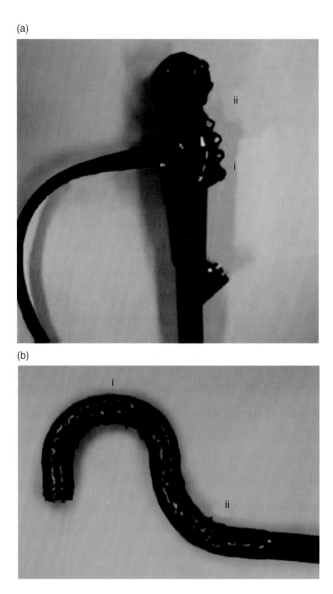

(b)

Fig. 15.1 (a) The operating section of the multibending scope (olympus XGIF-2T240M): (i) the up/down and right/left controls for the distal flexible portion; (ii) up/down control for the proximal flexible portion. (b) The outer diameter of the distal end of the M-scope, showing a sen-neck endoscopic tip: (i) the distal flexible portion; (ii) the proximal flexible portion.

be difficult to obtain with conventional endoscopes. Downward bending of the proximal section and upward bending of the distal section allows frontal viewing of lesions located on the lesser curvature. On the other hand, upward bending of the proximal section and downward bending of the distal section provides a frontal view of the lesion on a greater curvature.

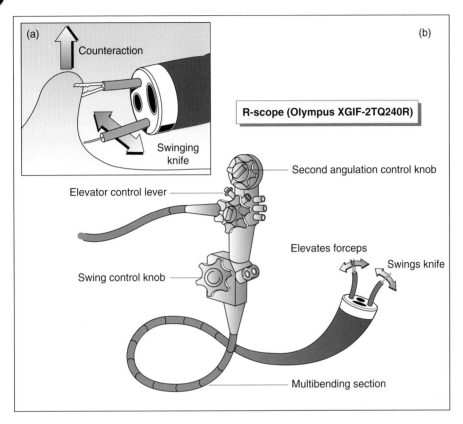

Fig. 15.2 (a) The grasping forceps lift the neoplastic lesion vertically, moving it up and away from the muscle layer for lesion counter traction, and an electrocautery knife swings horizontally to dissect the raised lesion. (b) The R-scope (XGIF-2TQ240R; Olympus Medical Systems, Tokyo, Japan) has two movable instrument channels: one moves vertically and the other swings horizontally. The two instruments can be manipulated during the operation with a knob and a lever that surround the angulation control knobs of the R-scope. Once the operator has decided on the knob or lever positions, these can easily be locked into position. The R-scope also has a multibending system.

Robotics endoscope ('R-scope')

A new therapeutic endoscope, the 'R-scope' (XGIF-2TQ240R; Olympus Medical Systems, Tokyo, Japan; Fig. 15.2(a),(b) is equipped with a multibending system and has two independently movable instrument channels: one can move a grasping forceps vertically for lesion counter-traction; the other can swing a cutting knife horizontally for dissection. Moreover, this new endoscope is equipped with a water-jet system for maintaining clear views even in hemorrhagic areas. Our study of ESD using the R-scope [2] demonstrated efficacy with minimal complications and has significantly shortened operation times when compared to conventional ESD.

Next steps toward the future

Endoscopic suturing technique

In order to minimize the complication rates in ESD, ideally it would be better to close the defect after resection. However at the moment there is no commercially available endoscopic device capable of suturing the gastrointestinal wall closed. There are several methods currently used to close the defect after EMR or ESD endoscopically. These include clip application [3] and clip application with subsequent endoloop placement to close the gap between the edges of a perforation.

The next paragraph discribes two prototypes for the endoscopic suturing technique.

Eagle Claw

The 'Eagle Claw' is a complex flexible endoscopic sewing machine with an unusual action. Although most surgical stitches, whether placed at open surgery or at laparoscopy, are delivered using a curved needle, this is the first flexible endoscopic sewing device that attempts to solve the difficulties of sewing using a curved needle. The proximal end of the thread is passed through a thread lock which is tightened using a pushing catheter passed through a channel in the device once the two stitches have been placed. This device has not yet been used in patients [4]. Pham AV *et al.* [5] have used this device for the closure of colon perforation in pigs and they reported good results. Another application of this device for a new endoscopic therapy such as NOTES is expected in future.

The next paragraph presents the new sewing method that has been developed by our group and might be useful for closing defects following ESD.

New sewing method using T-tags on thread and a locking and cutting device

This new sewing device has been developed and tested [6]. It has also been called a tissue approximation system or TAS. It is not yet commercially available although it is likely to become so in a few months time once it has FDA clearance and a CE mark. This device places a T-tag on a thread into tissue using a 20-gauge needle. Knots are tied by using a thread locking system. The suturing and knot locking can be accomplished through a 2.8 mm accessory channel in a conventional gastroscope (or colonoscope) and has also been used under endoscopic ultrasound guidance.

Endoscopic full-thickness resection (EFTR)

An effective and reliable endoscopic suturing device would allow full-thickness resection of the gastric wall for the treatment of early-stage cancer (Fig. 15.3).

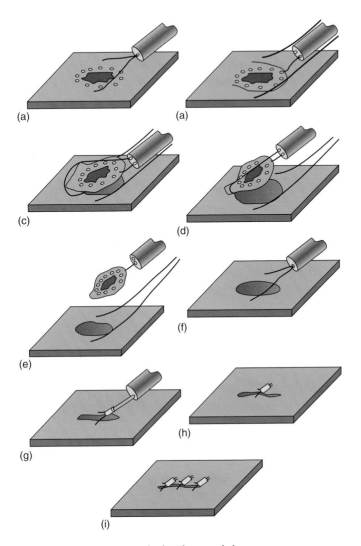

(a)

(a)

(c)

(d)

(e)

(f)

(g)

(h)

(i)

Fig. 15.3 Full-thickness resection method with sutured closure.

Endoscopic full-thickness resection would allow complete histopathological examination of the cancer and allow less invasive removal of more deeply penetrating cancers, which have not spread to the serosal surface [7]. We have described a method using an endoscopic variceal ligation (EVL) device [8] without prior injection of saline, and a bidirectional cutter without prior injection of saline. We have also reported a method of circumferential full-thickness excision with subsequent closure using an experimental bidirectional cutter [9]. The T-fastener method described above was applied in these studies to close the defect. They gave good results and were safe in studies on pigs.

Endoscopic mucosal resection device for Barrett's esophagus

We have described an experimental endoscopic resection device for Barrett's esophagus, which has an action similar to a potato peeler. The abnormal mucosa is sucked into a sling in an overtube, a small gauge needle is passed subcutaneously, and saline is used to separate the deep muscle from the submucosa and mucosa. A curved wire is used to slice long linear strips off the esophagus (Figs 15.4, 15.5, and 15.6).

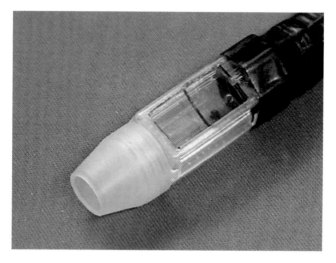

Fig. 15.4   Experimental Barrett's resection device.

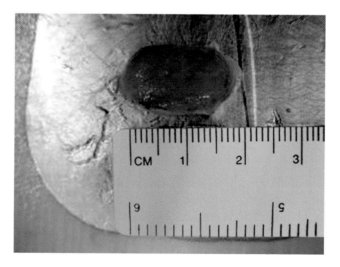

Fig. 15.5   Esophageal resection specimen.

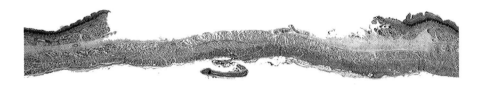

Fig. 15.6   Histology.

Perspectives for the future

There is room for improvement in EMR, ESD and full-thickness resection. Better ways to elevate and maintain a plane between the mucosa and submucosa under the lesion being resected would help. Better endoscopic control during cutting would be very useful – it is very easy to perforate the stomach and even easier to perforate the colon using needle knives. There is room for improvement in hemostasis and the development of bipolar forceps and more effective clips which can compress larger vessels and can be rotated, opened and closed on the vessel before firing are desirable and are likely to be available shortly. Because needle knives are relatively imprecise and because snares in end-caps can only take relatively small circular pieces of tissue, thus preventing en bloc resection, alternative approaches are needed. If EMR can only be performed safely and effectively by very skilled and experienced endoscopists who take a very long time per patient for endoscopy then it seems likely that there is room for innovation to make this less invasive surgical treatment of cancer easier, quicker and safer for less-skilled operators.

References

1 Sumiyama K, Kaise M, Nakayoshi T *et al.* Combined use of a magnifying endoscope with a narrow band imaging system and a multibending endoscope for en bloc EMR of early stage gastric cancer. *Gastrointest Endosc* 2004; **60**(1): 79–84.
2 Yonezawa J, Kaise M, Sumiyama K, Goda K, Arakawa H, Tajiri H. A novel double-channel therapeutic endoscope ('R-scope') facilitates endoscopic submucosal dissection of superficial gastric neoplasms. *Endoscopy* 2006; **38**(10): 1011–15.
3 Minami S, Gotoda T, Ono H, Oda I, Hamanaka H. Complete endoscopic closure of gastric perforation induced by endoscopic resection of early gastric cancer using endoclips can prevent surgery (with video). *Gastrointest Endosc* 2006; **63**(4): 602–5.
4 Hu B, Chung SC, Sun LC *et al.* Endoscopic suturing without extracorporeal knots: a laboratory study. *Gastrointest Endosc* 2005; **62**(2): 230–3.
5 Pham BV, Raju GS, Ahmed I *et al.* Immediate endoscopic closure of colon perforation by using a prototype endoscopic suturing device: feasibility and outcome in a porcine model (with video). *Gastrointest Endosc* 2006; **64**(1): 113–19.

6 Fritscher Ravens A, Mosse CA, Mills T, Park P-O, Mukherjee D, Swain P. A through-the-scope device for suturing and tissue approximation under endoscopic ultrasound control. *Gastrointestinal Endosc* 2002: **56(5):** 737–42.

7 Kantsevoy SV.Endoscopic full-thickness resection: new minimally invasive therapeutic alternative for GI-tract lesions. *Gastrointest Endosc* 2006; **64(1):** 90–1.

8 Ikeda K, Mosse CA, Park PO *et al.* Endoscopic full-thickness resection: circumferential cutting method. *Gastrointest Endosc* 2006; **64(1):** 82–9.

9 Ikeda K, Fritscher-Ravens A, Mosse CA, Mills T, Tajiri H, Swain CP. Endoscopic full-thickness resection with sutured closure in a porcine model. *Gastrointest Endosc* 2005; **62(1):** 122–9.

Index

Page numbers in **bold** refers to Tables and *italics* refers to Figures